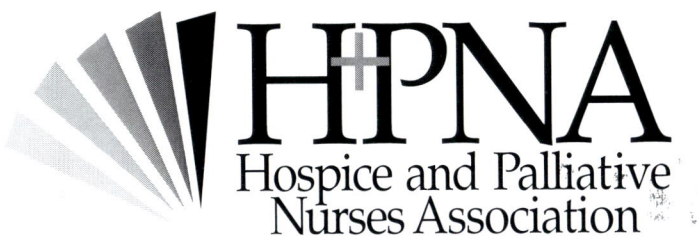

Core Curriculum for the Licensed Practical/Vocational Hospice and Palliative Nurse

Second Edition

Coordinating Editor:

Tami Borneman, RN, PHN, MSN, CNS, FPCN
Senior Research Specialist
Nursing Research and Education
City of Hope National Medical Center
Duarte, CA

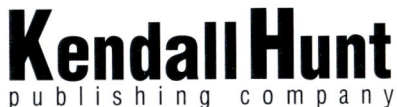

Kendall Hunt
publishing company

www.kendallhunt.com
Send all inquiries to:
4050 Westmark Drive
Dubuque, IA 52004-1840

Copyright © 2005, 2010 by Hospice and Palliative Nurses Association

ISBN 978-0-7575-7963-9

Kendall Hunt Publishing Company has the exclusive rights to reproduce this work, to prepare derivative works from this work, to publicly distribute this work, to publicly perform this work, and to publicly display this work.

All rights reserved. No part of this publication may be reproduced, stored in a retrieval system, or transmitted, in any form or by any means, electronic, mechanical, photocopying, recording, or otherwise, without the prior written permission of the copyright owner.

Printed in the United States of America
10　9　8　7　6　5　4　3　2　1

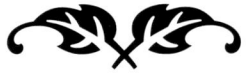

CONTENTS

CONTRIBUTORS ix

EXPERT REVIEWERS xi

DISCLAIMER xiii

INTRODUCTION xv

CHAPTER I: AN OVERVIEW OF HOSPICE AND PALLIATIVE CARE

I.	History of Hospice And Palliative Care	1
II.	Development of Modern Hospice and Palliative Care Movements	2
III.	Hospice Philosophy	4
IV.	Philosophy of Palliative Care	5

CHAPTER II: THE INTERDISCIPLINARY TEAM IN HOSPICE AND PALLIATIVE NURSING

I.	Introduction	11
II.	Collaboration of the IDT	13
III.	Team Leadership	13
IV.	Coordinated Decision-Making	14
V.	Conflict Resolution	14
VI.	LP/VN Roles in the Interdisciplinary Team	15
VII.	Additional Members of the Interdisciplinary Team	16
VIII.	Characteristics of a Well-Functioning Hospice and/or Palliative Care Team	16
IX.	Evaluation Process of the Interdisciplinary Team Functions	17

CHAPTER III: PATTERNS OF DISEASE PROGRESSION

I.	Cancer	21
II.	Treatment of Cancer	25
III.	Human Immunodeficiency Virus Infection (HIV Infection)	26
IV.	Acquired Immunodeficiency Syndrome (AIDS)	26

V.	Neurological Conditions	27
VI.	Cardiac Conditions	28
VII.	Pulmonary Diseases	28
VIII.	Kidney Diseases	29
IX.	General Debility	30
X.	Endocrine Diseases	31

CHAPTER IV: PAIN MANAGEMENT

I.	Introduction	35
II.	Assessment of Pain: effectiveness of pain management is directly related to assessment	37
III.	Pharmacologic Intervention	43
IV.	Pain during the Final Days of Life	49
V.	Summary of Principles of Pain Management	50
VI.	Evaluation: pain management is predicated by ongoing assessment of treatment efficacy and control of treatment side effects	51

CHAPTER V: SYMPTOM MANAGEMENT

I.	Principles	57
II.	Alteration in Skin and Mucous Membranes	58
III.	Altered Mental Status: Confusion, Delirium, Terminal Restlessness, Agitation	65
IV.	Anorexia and Cachexia	71
V.	Ascites	74
VI.	Aphasia	75
VII.	Bladder Spasms	77
VIII.	Bowel Incontinence	78
IX.	Bowel Obstruction	80
X.	Constipation	82
XI.	Diarrhea	85
XII.	Dysphagia/Odynophagia	87
XIII.	Dyspnea/Cough	89
XIV.	Edema	92
XV.	Extrapyramidal Symptoms (EPS)	93
XVI.	Hematologic Symptoms	95
XVII.	Hiccoughs	97

XVIII.	Impaired Mobility, Fatigue, Lethargy, Weakness	100
XIX.	Increased Intracranial Pressure (ICP)	103
XX.	Myoclonus	104
XXI.	Nausea and Vomiting	106
XXII.	Paresthesia and Neuropathy	110
XXIII.	Seizures	112
XXIV.	Urinary Incontinence/Retention	114

CHAPTER VI: COMMUNICATING AT THE END OF LIFE

I.	Basic Concepts of Communication	121
II.	Elements of Therapeutic Communication: Special Issues in Working with the Dying	124
III.	Dealing with Conflict	129

CHAPTER VII: CULTURAL CONSIDERATIONS IN END-OF-LIFE CARE

I.	Culture	133
II.	Cultural Sensitivity and Cultural Competence	135
III.	Cultural Values in the United States	136
IV.	Models for Cultural Assessment	136
V.	Culture and End of Life	139
VI.	Culture and End-of-Life Decision-Making	140
VII.	Selected Multicultural Views of End-of-Life Decisions	141
VIII.	Culture and End-of-Life Symptom Management	141
IX.	Cultural Responses to Death and Death Rituals	142
X.	Cultural Response to Death: Grief and Mourning	143
XI.	Summary	144

CHAPTER VIII: SPIRITUAL CARE AT THE END OF LIFE

I.	Definitions	147
II.	Importance of Spiritual Care in Palliative Care	148
III.	Spiritual Needs of the Dying Patient	148
IV.	Fears or Concerns of the Dying Patient Related to Spirituality	149
V.	Questions Patients Might Ask That Indicate a Spiritual Need or Concern	149
VI.	Spiritual Signs That Death Is Coming Soon	150

VII.	Common Religious/Spiritual Views on Death and Death Rituals	150
VIII.	Spiritual Interventions (Actions) of the Licensed Practical/Vocational Nurse	152
IX.	Summary	154

Chapter IX: End-of-Life Care for the Child and Family

I.	Introduction	157
II.	Common Pediatric Diagnoses Seen in Palliative and Hospice Care	157
III.	Differences between Pediatric and Adult Hospice Care	162
IV.	General Issues Related to Admission of Pediatric Patients	163
V.	Developmental Considerations in Pediatric Assessment	166
VI.	General Care Issues for Child/Family	168
VII.	Counsel/Provide Emotional Support for Child's Grief	172

Chapter X: Family Caregivers

I.	Recognizing Roles/Needs of Family Caregivers at the End of Life	179
II.	Physical Concerns of Family Caregivers	180
III.	Emotional Needs of Family Caregivers	180
IV.	Roles and Relationship Needs/Issues	181
V.	Spiritual Concerns	182

Chapter XI: Bereavement

I.	Introduction: Definitions	187
II.	Stages/Process of Grief	187
III.	Assessment	189
IV.	Interventions/Resources	190
V.	Recognition of Staff Grief	192
VI.	Conclusion	194

Chapter XII: Care at the Time of Dying

I.	Introduction/Overview	197
II.	Patient and Family Needs and Goals Related to the Dying Process	198
III.	The Environment	199
IV.	Symptom Management Related to Decline in Status	200
V.	Psychosocial and Spiritual Issues	204

VI.	Death	207
VII.	Professional Caregiver Coping with Care of the Dying	209
VIII.	Conclusion	209

CHAPTER XIII: PERSONAL AND PROFESSIONAL DEVELOPMENT

I.	Introduction	211
II.	Definitions	211
III.	Professional Expectations and Development	216
IV.	Addressing Professional Stresses	219

APPENDIX 1: WEBSITE/INTERNET RESOURCES	223
APPENDIX 2: COMMONLY USED MEDICATIONS	227

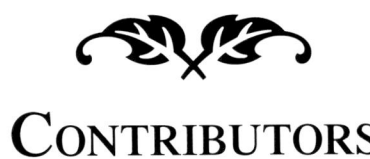

CONTRIBUTORS

Tami Borneman, RN, PHN, MSN, CNS, FPCN
Senior Research Specialist
Nursing Research and Education
City of Hope National Medical Center
Duarte, CA

Mary Ersek, PhD, RN, FAAN, FPCN
Associate Director, John A. Hartford Center
 of Geriatric Nursing Excellence and Center
 for Integrative Science in Aging
Associate Professor
University of Pennsylvania School of Nursing
Philadelphia, PA

Linda M. Gorman, RN, MN, PMHCNS-BC
Palliative Care Clinical Nurse Specialist
Cedars-Sinai Medical Center
Los Angeles, CA

Lynda Gruenwald-Schmitz, RN, MSN, CHPN®
Aurora VNA Zilber Family Hospice
Wauwatosa, WI

Barbara Anderson Head, PhD, RN, CHPN®,
 ACSW
Assistant Professor
Interdisciplinary Program for Palliative Care
 and Chronic Illness
University of Louisville School of Medicine
Louisville, KY

Beth Miller Kraybill, BSN, CHPN® MDiv.
Seattle Mennonite Church
Seattle WA

Judy Lentz, RN, MSN, NHA
Chief Executive Officer
Hospice and Palliative Nurses Association
Pittsburgh, PA

Jeanne Martinez, RN, MPH, CHPN®, FPCN
Quality and Education Specialist
Northwestern Memorial Home Health Care
Chicago, IL

Marianne Matzo, PhD, GNP-BC, FPCN, FAAN
Professor and Frances E. and A. Earl Ziegler Chair
 in Palliative Care Nursing
University of Oklahoma Health Sciences Center
 College
Oklahoma City, OK

Beverly Paukstis, RN, MS, CHPN®, CHPA®
Director of Hospice Operations
The Washington Home and Community Hospices
 of DC, VA, MD
Washington, DC

Marty Richards, MSW, LICSW
Social Worker
Private Practice
Port Townsend, WA

Roger Strong, PhD, RN, ACHNP®, FPCN
Nurse Practitioner
San Diego Hospice
San Diego, CA

Dena Jean Sutermaster, RN, MSN, CHPN®
Director of Education Products
Hospice and Palliative Nurses Association
Pittsburgh, PA

Christy Torkildson, RN, PHN, MSN
Lead Faculty
Unitek College, Department of Nursing
　Consultant, Pediatric Palliative Care
Doctoral Student, University of California
　San Francisco School of Nursing
San Ramon, CA

Sarah A. Wilson, PhD, RN
Associate Professor
Director, Institute for End-of-Life Care Education
Marquette University
Milwaukee, WI

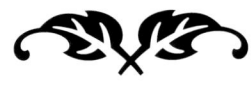

EXPERT REVIEWERS

Elmar Aroma, LVN
Staff, Odyssey Hospice of Northern California
Hayward, CA

Tami Borneman, RN, PHN, MSN, CNS, FPCN
Senior Research Specialist
Nursing Research and Education
City of Hope National Medical Center
Duarte, CA

Carma Erickson-Hurt, APRN, ACHPN
Faculty
Grand Canyon University
Phoenix, AZ

Nancy L. Grandovic, RN, BSN, MEd., CHPN®
Director of Education Services
Hospice and Palliative Nurses Association
Pittsburgh, PA

Lisa Medeiros, BS, LVN
Staff, George Mark Children's House
San Leandro, CA

Dena Jean Sutermaster, RN, MSN, CHPN®
Director of Education Products
Hospice and Palliative Nurses Association
Pittsburgh, PA

Joseph C. Torkildson, MD, MBA
Director of Neuro-Oncology
Director of Inpatient Services
Department of Pediatric Hematology-Oncology
Children's Hospital and Research Center
Oakland, CA

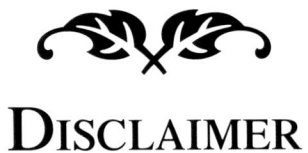

Disclaimer

The Hospice and Palliative Nurses Association,
its officers and directors and the authors and reviewers of this Core Curriculum
make no claims that buying or studying it will guarantee a passing score
on the CHPLN® Certification examination.

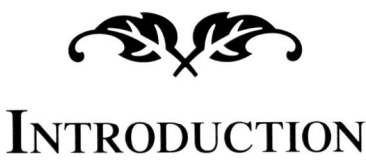

INTRODUCTION

Working in many settings, including long-term care, hospitals, and home care and hospice, licensed practical/vocational nurses play a central role in providing care to very sick and/or dying patients and their families. The cornerstone of their practice is the provision of evidence-based physical, emotional, psychosocial, and spiritual care in collaboration with the family, RN, and other members of the healthcare team. Because of their consistent interaction with the patients and families, LP/VNs are well positioned to observe the physical and psychosocial symptoms that are common to those who are very sick and/or terminal. They also see first hand the existential and spiritual issues with which the patients and their families struggle. They regularly witness and experience the profound, multiple losses, and grief that accompany the dying process.

The purpose of the *Core Curriculum for the Licensed Practical/Vocational Hospice and Palliative Nurse* is to recognize the LP/VN's role in palliative and end-of-life care, and to ensure adequate preparation and educational support for their work.

We realized that one of our biggest challenges was to address the diversity among LP/VNs. Practice and expertise differ based on geographic area and clinical setting, as well as the individual's cultural, educational, and experiential background. To help you understand how we incorporated these variations and made decisions about the depth and breadth of information, we want to make explicit the principles that guided the development of the *Core Curriculum*. We believe that:

- Better educational preparation for LP/VNs results in more effective care to dying patients and their families.

- LP/VNs are integral members of the hospice and palliative care team. In order to participate actively in planning and providing quality end-of-life care, they need to possess a thorough knowledge of hospice and palliative care concepts and practices.

- LP/VNs who are educated and involved in the care of dying patients experience greater job satisfaction, which may in turn decrease job turnover that threatens the quality and consistency of end-of-life care.

- LP/VNs do not make decisions about medical therapies; however they are to "demonstrate decision-making in the care of patients and families experiencing life-limiting, progressive illness through use of the nursing process to address the physical, emotional, psychosocial, and spiritual needs of the patients and families."[1,p1] In addition, their attitudes towards certain therapies, such as opioids and artificial nutrition, are communicated either directly or indirectly to patients and families. Thus, they need to be aware of the reasons for instituting or withdrawing therapies and to realize that their attitudes influence patients and families. For this reason, the *Core Curriculum for the Licensed Practical/Vocational Hospice and Palliative Nurse* contains information about medical therapies for several symptoms.

- Our goal is to ensure competent, professional end-of-life care. We understand that the knowledge and skill level suggested by some of the content may exceed your scope of practice in some settings. However, we present these materials to set the standard. Our experience as clinicians, educators, and researchers has shown us that many LP/VN's are deeply committed to their work and want to provide a high level of end-of-life care, not merely the minimum. This *Core Curriculum* was developed to reflect this goal.

The 2nd edition of this review manual is authored by credible experts from the field of hospice and palliative care. It has been reviewed by experts in these fields as well. This Core Curriculum is recognized as one of many excellent resources to be used in preparing for professional assessment activities. As you read through the chapters, please remember that you are to "reflect the scope and standards of hospice and palliative care under the direction of a registered nurse"[2,p7] as put forth in the *Statement on the Scope and Standards of Hospice and Palliative Licensed Practical/Vocational Nursing Practice*.

There are thirteen chapters covering: 1) Overview of Hospice and Palliative Care, 2) Interdisciplinary Collaboration, 3) Patterns of Disease Progression, 4) Pain, 5) Other Symptoms, 6) Communication, 7) Culture, 8) Spirituality, 9) Pediatrics, 10) Family Caregivers, 11) Loss and Bereavement, 12) Time of Death: Indicators of Imminent Death, and 13) Personal and Professional Development.

The scope of this project necessitates much help thereby warranting many "thank you's." We are very grateful to all of the contributing authors who willingly gave of their time and expertise, as well as the reviewers for their hard work. A special thank you to Judy Lentz, CEO of HPNA her support of this project.

Tami Borncman, RN, PHN, MSN, CNS, FPCN
Dena Jean Sutermaster, RN, MSN, CHPN®

CITED REFERENCES

1. Dahlin C, Lentz J, Sutermaster DJ. *Professional Competencies for the Hospice and Palliative Licensed Practical/Vocational Nurse*. Dubuque, IA: Kendall Hunt Publishing; 2004.
2. Dahlin C, Lentz J, Sutermaster DJ. *Statement of the Scope and Standards of Hospice and Palliative Licensed Practical/Vocational Nursing Practice*. Dubuque, IA: Kendall Hunt Publishing; 2004.

CHAPTER I

AN OVERVIEW OF HOSPICE AND PALLIATIVE CARE

Tami Borneman, RN, PHN, MSN, CNS, FPCN

Adapted from: Volker BG, Watson AC. An overview of hospice and palliative care. *Core Curriculum for the Hospice and Palliative Nurse*. 2nd ed. Dubuque, IA: Kendall Hunt Publishing; 2005.

I. **History of Hospice and Palliative Care**

   A. **Hospice**

   1. Concept antedates 475 AD

   2. The term "hospes," from which the term hospice is derived, means to be both host and guest; implies an interaction and mutual caring between patient, family, and hospice staff

   3. Self-sustained communities evolved after 335 AD where ill, weary, homeless, and dying persons received care

   4. During the early middle ages, words *hospice, hospital,* and *hostel* were used interchangeably

   5. Also during the middle ages *hospitia,* or traveler's rests provided food, shelter, as well as care for those sick or dying

   6. The care and support of the whole person (the soul, mind, spirit) evolved in these early hospices

   7. Evolved to care for the sick and incurables in 1800's

   8. The word hospice became synonymous with care of the terminally ill late in the 1800's with the founding of Our Lady's Hospice in Dublin by Sister May Aikenhead of the Irish Sisters of Charity, who was a colleague of Florence Nightingale

   9. St. Joseph's Hospice established in 1900 in London; Dame Cicely Saunders began refining the ideas and protocols that formed the cornerstone of modern hospice care in the 1950's and 60's

   10. Cicely Saunders, MD opened St. Christopher's Hospice in the 1960's in suburban London, marking the beginning of the modern hospice movement

   11. Cicely Saunders, MD visited the United States in 1963 and spoke to the medical and nursing students, and interested others at Yale University

12. Florence Wald, Dean of Yale School of Nursing, resigned to plan and found the Connecticut Hospice
13. The Palliative Care service at the Royal Victoria Hospital, Montreal, Canada, started by Balfour Mount, MD opened in 1975; first use of the term "palliative care" to refer to a program of care for terminally ill persons and their families; this became the first hospice in North America
14. The Connecticut Hospice incorporated in 1971, began seeing home care patients in 1974, 44 bed inpatient facility opened in 1979; the first hospice in the United States
15. 1983 Tax Equity Fiscal Responsibility Act created the Medicare Hospice Benefit; defines hospice care in the United States

B. Palliative Care

1. David Tasma, a Polish Jew who died of cancer in a London hospital in 1948 left Cicely Saunders a small legacy, saying, "I want to be a window in your home"
2. She acknowledges her interaction with him as the beginning of her work with thousands of dying patients, from which she established science of palliative medicine
    a) Attends to the whole person
    b) Is limited to those who have progressive predictable disease
    c) Uses scientific rigor in developing treatment for pain and symptoms[1]
3. Contrasting views exist about the evolution of palliative care
    a) Hospice and palliative care are often seen as synonymous (e.g., in England and Canada, hospice is also called palliative care)[2]
    b) Hospice is thought to be a subset of palliative care[3]
    c) Palliative care found its roots in hospice[4]

C. Hospice includes the elements of palliative care, but not all palliative care includes all the elements of hospice care[5]

II. Development of Modern Hospice and Palliative Care Movements

A. Hospice Landmark Events

1. Development of current concepts of palliative care are, in large part, through the work of Dame Cicely Saunders at St. Christopher's Hospice in London, including the use of scheduled oral opioids for pain management
2. Elisabeth Kübler-Ross's work in the 1960's demystified death and dying and opened the debate on care of the dying for healthcare professionals and the lay public; *On Death and Dying* was published in 1969
3. Increased knowledge and research regarding grief, loss, and bereavement
4. General dissatisfaction (among the public and some factions of the healthcare system) about how dying persons and their families are treated in the U.S. healthcare system which generally emphasizes technological intervention and over treatment to prevent death

5. Development of the holistic nursing practice model
6. Issues related to cost of care versus quality of life
7. Physician assisted suicide movement and the 1995 results of the SUPPORT study, showing high incidence of uncontrolled pain (from 74% to 95%) in very ill and dying adults in spite of planned interventions from nurses to encourage physicians to attend to pain control[6]
8. The "natural death" consumer movement similar to the natural childbirth movement
9. Publication by the National Hospice Organization (NHO) of *A Pathway for Patients and Families Facing Terminal Illness* (1997)
10. Development by the National Hospice and Palliative Care Organization (NHPCO) of *Hospice Standards of Practice* (2001)

B. Palliative Care

1. Major factors have influenced the recent development of palliative care programs in the United States

    a) Consumer demand

    (1) Aging of the population

    (2) Growing public interest in assisted suicide and euthanasia

    (3) Growing gap between what people with life-threatening illness desire and what they experience from healthcare systems and providers

    (4) Supreme Court's ruling on the right to die and its affirmation of right to care at the end of life

    b) Acknowledgment by medical community that care of dying is poor

    (1) SUPPORT Study results[6]

    (2) 1997 Institute of Medicine's report on End-of-life Care[7]

    (3) Development of WHO Standards for Cancer Pain Relief (1996)[8]

    (4) 1990 WHO guidelines on Cancer Pain Relief and Palliative Care[8]

    (5) AHCPR Cancer Pain Guidelines (now Agency for Healthcare Research and Quality [AHRQ])[9]

    (6) Grassroots development of State Cancer Pain Initiatives (now American Alliance of Cancer Pain Initiatives)

    (7) Efforts of Project on Death in America, LAST ACTS Initiative, and Center to Improve the Care of the Dying[10]

    (8) Americans for Better Care of the Dying (ABCD)

    (9) Center to Advance Palliative Care (CAPC)

    (10) The Joint Commission includes pain assessment and management as a part of the accreditation process for hospitals, home health, long-term care, long-term care pharmacies, ambulatory care, behavioral health, managed behavioral health, healthcare networks[11]

    (11) National Consensus Project *Clinical Practice Guidelines for Quality Palliative Care*

III. Hospice Philosophy

A. Definitions of Hospice

1. Medicare describes hospice as an approach to caring for terminally ill individuals that stresses palliative care (relief of pain and uncomfortable symptoms), as opposed to curative care. In addition to meeting the patient's medical needs, hospice care addresses the physical, psychosocial, and spiritual needs of the patient, as well as the psychosocial needs of the patient's family/caregiver. The emphasis of the hospice program is on keeping the hospice patient at home with family and friends as long as possible

2. The National Hospice and Palliative Care Organization (NHPCO) describes hospice as a specialized form of multidisciplinary healthcare, which is designed to provide palliative care, alleviate the physical, emotional, social, and spiritual discomforts of an individual who is experiencing the last phase of life due to the existence of a life-limiting, progressive disease, to provide supportive care to the primary caregiver and the family of the hospice patient

3. Hospice and Palliative Nurses Association (HPNA) defines hospice nursing as the provision of palliative nursing care for the terminally ill and their families with the emphasis on their physical, psychosocial, emotional, and spiritual needs. This care is accomplished in collaboration with an interdisciplinary team through a service that is available 24 hours a day, 7 days a week. The service comprises pain and symptom management, bereavement and volunteer components. Hospice nursing, then, is holistic practice conducted within an affiliated matrix. The hospice nurse, in developing and maintaining collaborative relationships with other members of the interdisciplinary team, must be flexible in dealing with the inevitable role blending that takes place. In functioning as a case manager, coordinating the implementation of the interdisciplinary team developed plan of care, the hospice nurse also shares an advocacy role for patients and their families with other members of the team

B. Key Concepts in Hospice Philosophy

1. The patient and family (as defined by the patient) are considered the single unit of care

2. Hospice uses a core interdisciplinary team to address the physical, social, emotional, and spiritual needs of the patient and family

3. Hospice provides for the medical treatment of pain and other distressing symptoms associated with the life-limiting, progressive illness, but does not provide interventions to cure the disease or prolong life

4. The interdisciplinary team develops the overall plan of care, in accordance with the wishes of the patient and family, in order to provide coordinated care that emphasizes supportive services such as home care, pain management, and limited inpatient services

5. Hospice care actively engages the community by utilizing volunteer support in delivering hospice services

6. The patient's home, or place of primary residence no matter where that may be (skilled nursing or residential care facilities, prisons, shelters, daycare centers for the elderly, etc.), is the primary site of hospice care

7. The philosophy of hospice emphasizes comfort, dignity and quality of life, with the focus on spiritual and existential issues throughout dying, death, and bereavement

8. Patients and families are empowered to achieve as much control over their lives as possible

C. **Desired Goals for End-of-Life Care**[12]

1. Self-determined life closure: terminally ill patients who are mentally competent should have freedom to decide how the rest of their life is spent within the options allowed by law

2. Safe and comfortable dying: patients are able to die free of distressing symptoms

3. Effective grieving: surviving family members/significant others are supported through the normal grieving process

D. **Issues for Hospice**

1. Six months life expectancy (should the disease run its usual course) or less may be seen as death sentence by some physicians who thus may be reluctant to refer to hospice

2. Insurers may not pay for high-tech care and may limit access to specialists

3. Physicians may be reluctant to discuss Do Not Resuscitate (DNR) orders; patient and family may not be ready to accept them although DNR orders are not required for hospice admission

4. Referrals often occur when death is imminent, thus rushing hospice to quickly bond with family and initiate symptom management in crisis mode

5. Significant barriers to the management of pain continue to exist (see Chapter IV)

6. Compliance with the Centers for Medicare and Medicaid Service's Conditions of Participation

IV. **Philosophy of Palliative Care**

A. **Definitions of Palliative Care**

1. The National Consensus Project[13] defines palliative care as

a) The goal of palliative care is to prevent and relieve suffering and to support the best possible quality of life for patients and their families, regardless of the stage of the disease or the need for other therapies. Palliative care is both a philosophy of care and an organized, highly structured system for delivering care. Palliative care expands traditional disease-model medical treatments to include the goals of enhancing quality of life for patient and family, optimizing function, helping with decision-making, and providing opportunities for personal growth. As such, it can be delivered concurrently with life-prolonging care or as the main focus of care

b) Palliative care is operationalized through effective management of pain and other distressing symptoms, while incorporating psychosocial and spiritual care with consideration of patient and family needs, preferences, values, beliefs, and culture. Evaluation and treatment should be comprehensive and patient-centered with a focus on the central role of the family unit in decision-making. Palliative care affirms life by supporting the patient and family's goals for the future, including their hopes for cure or life-prolongation, as well as their hopes for peace and dignity throughout the course of illness, the dying process, and death. Palliative care aims to guide and assist the patient and family in making decisions that enable them to work toward their goals during whatever time they have remaining. Comprehensive palliative care services often require the expertise of various providers to adequately assess and treat the complex needs of seriously ill patients and their families. Leadership, collaboration, coordination, and communication are key elements for effective integration of these disciplines and services

2. World Health Organization defines palliative care as an approach to care, which improves quality of life of patients and their families facing life-threatening illness, through the prevention and relief of suffering by means of early identification and impeccable assessment and treatment of pain and other problems, physical, psychological, and spiritual[14]

3. Palliative care is defined as ". . . the prevention and relief of suffering through the management of symptoms from the early through the final stages of an illness" and ". . . attends closely to the emotional, spiritual, and practical needs/goals of the patient and family with life-threatening disease across the illness, dying trajectory" by the Institute of Medicine Task Force[7]

B. **Key Concepts of Palliative Care Philosophy**[15]

1. Affirms life and regards dying as a normal process that is neither hastened nor postponed

2. Provides relief from pain and other distressing symptoms

3. Integrates the psychological and spiritual aspects of patient care

4. Offers a support system to help the family cope during the patient's illness and their own bereavement

C. **Precepts of Palliative Care According to the Last Acts Initiative,**[16] **1998**

1. Respect for patient goals, preferences, and choices

2. Comprehensive care

   a) Addresses holistic needs

   b) Alleviates isolation

   c) Commits to ongoing communication and non-abandonment

3. Utilizes strengths of interdisciplinary resources

4. Acknowledges/addresses caregiver concerns and desire for supportive services

5. Develops institutional infrastructures that support best practices and best models of palliative care

6. Excellent interdisciplinary team coordination among all caregiving environments

7. Focus of care based on patient and family values, addresses holistic growth and healing

8. Care is flexible (e.g., curative, palliative, or preventive in focus)

D. **Core Principles of Palliative Care**

1. Family is the unit of care

2. Meaning of disease, suffering, life, and death are addressed within each unique family unit

3. Commitment to collaboration through team process

4. Ethical principles of care are incorporated into daily practice

E. **Issues for Palliative Care**
 1. Patients, families and staff may have difficulty transitioning from curative to palliative care
 2. Most programs are located in hospital-based, hierarchical medical institutions
 3. Some programs may not provide continuity and communication with primary care physicians and community-based programs
 4. Some programs may not provide supportive services, such as social work, spiritual, volunteer or bereavement follow-up

Cited References

1. Conner SR. New initiatives transforming hospice care. *The Hospice Journal.* 1999;14(3/4):193–203.
2. O'Connor P. Hospice vs. palliative care. *The Hospice Journal.* 1999;14(3/4):123–137.
3. Byock IR. Hospice and palliative care: a parting of the ways or a path to the future. *Journal of Palliative Medicine.* 1998;1:165–176.
4. Portenoy PR. *Defining Palliative Care.* Beth Israel Medical Center: Newsletter, Department of Pain and Palliative Care; 1998.
5. Brenner R. Hospice care and palliative care: a perspective from experience. *The Hospice Journal.* 1999;14(3/4):155–166.
6. The SUPPORT Principal Investigators. A controlled trial to improve care for seriously ill patients. *JAMA.* 1995;274:1591–1598.
7. Field MJ, Cassel CK. *Approaching Death: Improving Care at the End of Life.* Washington, DC: Institute of Medicine Task Force; 1997.
8. World Health Organization (WHO). Report of a WHO Expert Committee. *Cancer Pain Relief and Palliative Care.* WHO Technical Support Series, No. 804. Geneva: World Health Organization; 1986, 1990, 1996.
9. Jacox A, Carr DB, Payne R, et al. *Management of Cancer Pain. Clinical Practice Guideline.* No. 9. AHCPR Publication No. 94-0592. Rockville, MD: Agency for Health Care Policy and Research, U.S. Department of Health and Human Services, Public Health Service; March 1994.
10. Bookbinder M, McHugh M. Societal perspectives regarding palliative care. In: Matzo M, Sherman DW, eds. *Palliative Care Nursing: Quality Care to the End of Life.* 3rd ed. New York, NY: Springer Publishing; 2010:75–95.
11. The Joint Commission. *The Joint Commission Requirements.* Available at: www.jointcommission.org. Accessed February 2, 2010.
12. National Hospice Organization. *A Pathway for Patients and Families Facing Terminal Illness.* Arlington, VA: National Hospice Organization; 1997:5–6.
13. National Consensus Project for Quality Palliative Care. *Clinical Practice Guidelines for Quality Palliative Care.* 2nd ed. 2009. Available at: www.nationalconsensusproject.org. Accessed February 2, 2010.
14. World Health Organization. *National Cancer Control Programs: Policies and Managerial Guidelines.* 2nd ed. 2002.
15. Storey P, Knight CF. *Hospice/Palliative Care Training For Physicians (UNIPACS 2, 2, 4, 6).* 3rd ed. Chicago, IL: American Academy of Hospice and Palliative Medicine; 2008.
16. Task Force on Palliative Care. Last acts: precepts of palliative care. 1997. Available at: www.aacn.org/WD/Palliative/Docs/2001Precep.pdf. Accessed May 27, 2010.

ADDITIONAL REFERENCES AND RESOURCES

Abu-Saad HH. Palliative care: an international view. *Patient Education and Counseling.* 2000;41:15–22.

Ferrell BR, Coyle N, eds. *Textbook of Palliative Nursing.* 3rd ed. New York, NY: Oxford University Press; 2010.

Krisman-Scott MA. Origins of hospice in the United States: the care of the dying, 1945–1975. *Journal of Hospice and Palliative Nursing.* 2002;5(4):205–210.

National Hospice and Palliative Care Organization. *Facts and Figures on Hospice Care in America.* Washington, DC: National Hospice and Palliative Care Organization; 2008. Available at: www.nhpco.org/files/public/Statistics_Research/NHPCO_facts-and-figures_2008.pdf

Payne SK, Smith TJ, Coyne P, et al. *A High Volume Specialist Palliative Care Unit (PCU) and Team Reduces End of Life (EOL) Costs* [ASCO abstract 2001]. American Society of Clinical Oncology. Available at: www.asco.org/ASCOv2/Meetings/Abstracts?&vmview=abst_detail_view&confID=10&abstractID=1556. Accessed May 2010.

Saunders C. The evolution of palliative care. *Patient Education and Counseling.* [abstract taken from Patient Education and Counseling]; Am J Med. 2000;(41):7–13. Available at: http://www.pec-journal.com/article/S0738-3991(00)0010-5/abstract. Accessed on May 2010.

Chapter II

The Interdisciplinary Team in Hospice and Palliative Nursing

Linda M. Gorman, RN, MN, PMHCNS-BC

I. **Introduction**

  A. **The Interdisciplinary Team (IDT)**

   1. The interdisciplinary team is a group of individuals with varied and specialized training who collaborate to coordinate their activities to provide services for clients

   2. In hospice and/or palliative care the IDT usually consists of the professionals and nonprofessionals who are involved in the care of the patient and his/her family

   3. The complex physical, psychosocial, spiritual, and bereavement issues facing the patient and his/her family receiving hospice and palliative care requires professionals with a broad range of knowledge[1-3]

   4. Because of the complex and multidimensional needs of seriously ill and terminally ill patients, the interdisciplinary team in hospice and palliative care is essential[1-2]

   5. No one professional can address all the complex needs of these patients/families so working with a group of team members representing multiple disciplines ensures that the varied needs can be met more effectively

   6. A strength of the team is that each member has a unique view of the patient and family[3]

   7. In hospice, core team members required by hospice regulations include

      a) Hospice physician

      b) RN case manager

      c) Social worker

      d) Counselor

   8. Other hospice team members may include other nurses, hospice aides, volunteers, pharmacists, chaplains, bereavement coordinators, dietitians, psychologists, and therapists, amongst others

9. Palliative care interdisciplinary team membership is more varied but can include the following[4]
    a) Core group of professionals should include medicine, nursing (including advanced practice nurses), and social work
    b) Others may include some combination of the following
        (1) Volunteer coordinators
        (2) Dietitians
        (3) Nursing assistants
        (4) Pharmacists
        (5) Chaplains
        (6) Bereavement coordinators
        (7) Psychologists
        (8) Therapists (physical, occupations, art, play music, child-life)
        (9) Case managers
        (10) Trained volunteers
    c) Strong team members are vital to the success of a palliative care program[2]
10. Each member of the team has a unique view of the patient and family[3]
11. Important components of the interdisciplinary team[1]
    a) Collaboration
    b) Patient and family-directed goal setting
    c) Interdisciplinary planning of interventions
12. The key to effective interdisciplinary team functioning includes collaboration, leadership, coordinated decision-making, and conflict resolution[3]

B. Multidisciplinary Team
1. In the traditional multidisciplinary approach, members representing each discipline independently formulate goals based on their own area of expertise[5]
2. The group may meet but independent plans from each discipline are developed
3. In other models the group may only communicate through the medical record rather than meeting face to face
4. The physician is often the team leader in a traditional multidisciplinary team[3]
5. This model is often utilized in the acute hospital setting
6. The multidisciplinary team is not utilized in the hospice/palliative care setting

II. Collaboration of the IDT

A. Characteristics of Effective Collaboration[3,6]

1. Assessment data is shared so all disciplines have the same information
2. All members participate in development of the plan of care
3. Information is utilized in accordance with the expressed needs and wishes of the patient and family
4. Shared planning, decision-making, accountability, and responsibility for the care of the patient are implied in the interdisciplinary team
5. Collaboration implies that team members are aware of each other's roles. This can be accomplished by
    a) Joint visits so disciplines can understand each other's contributions
    b) Educating team members of role functions
    c) All team members respect and attend to assessments and contributions made by each other
    d) Team members understand their own role in the team and appreciation of the contribution of other members is fostered
6. Team members must collaborate with other healthcare professionals essential to the patient's care who may not be part of the interdisciplinary team (e.g., primary physician, psychotherapist, nurse practitioner from the community)
7. Decisions are made after all information has been gathered and all team members contribute
8. Remaining clear on the goals for the patient and family should drive all decisions rather than one team member's perspective
9. Collaboration builds interdisciplinary awareness of interdependence of the team[1]

III. Team Leadership

A. Designating the Team Leader

1. Though one individual may be designated as the leader, all members share responsibility to participate and contribute
2. The team leader may be any member of the team

B. Characteristics of an Effective Leader of an Interdisciplinary Team Include[6]

1. Promotes collaboration and communication
2. Encourages input from all members of the team
3. Recognizes when conflict is occurring and works with whole team to address
4. Recognizes need to complete tasks within set time-frame and works with group to accomplish this
5. Supports diverse opinions and new ideas to be introduced to the group

IV. Coordinated Decision-Making

A. Team members incorporate each discipline's assessment of the patient and family into the comprehensive plan of care[1]

B. Care goals are based on team member assessments and patient and family needs and wishes

C. Other healthcare providers who are not part of the team will be incorporated as needed

D. Team members discuss complex situations so all information is gathered before difficult decisions are made

E. The plan of care is systematically updated on a regular basis to ensure goals defined by the patient and family are being addressed and continuity of care is maintained

V. Conflict Resolution[6-7]

A. Communication is the foundation of all team functioning

B. Conflict tends to arise when there are barriers to effective communication

C. Conflict is expected to occur since members are interdependent on each other

D. Team members need to feel they are equals and that each can offer ideas and recommendations on ways to improve team functioning

E. Factors that may contribute to conflict within the team include
   1. Ambiguous role boundaries
   2. Communication barriers
   3. Leadership style that is not appropriate for the situation or congruent with the team's needs
   4. Team members with differing goals and expectations
   5. Poorly stated purpose of the meeting
   6. Lack of training in interdisciplinary collaboration
   7. Group that is too large or too small for the stated purpose
   8. Poor mechanisms to achieve timely exchange of information

F. **Types of conflict**
   1. Intrapersonal: team members may have conflicting feelings with a colleague
   2. Interpersonal: recurring differences between team members with different personality styles

3. Intragroup: subgroups within a team that are in conflict with other subgroups
4. Intergroup: conflict between programs or other teams

G. **Preventing team conflict**
1. Self awareness within team of potential conflict areas
2. Reviewing decisions when disagreement is evident
3. Examination of overlapping roles and considering renegotiation of roles and assignments
4. Recognize professional hierarchies exist and discuss openly (e.g., some member(s) tend to defer to an experienced, well respected physician)
5. Team building exercises
6. Develop ground rules
7. Encourage open environment to discuss disagreements
8. Invite other professionals to the team meeting and encourage their input
9. Develop an evaluation process of team functioning that is accomplished periodically
10. Analyze retention rates and satisfaction levels of members

H. **Addressing team conflict**
1. Most important is to recognize team conflict and not ignore it
2. Brainstorm possible solutions with whole team
3. Separate the person from the problem (e.g., avoid focusing on an individual's personality trait that irritates some members). Rather focus on how the trait impacts communication
4. Use objective criteria when possible
5. Seek outside consultation with organizational development professionals when needed
6. Support constructive and respectful criticism
7. Identify areas of agreement
8. Remember that the presence of conflict can often bring growth and potential for change and should not be avoided[3]

VI. **LP/VN Roles in the Interdisciplinary Team**[8-9]

A. **The LP/VN plays an important role in the IDT**
1. Communicate information from systematic data collection of the multidimensional aspects of the needs of the patients and family
2. Collaborate with other members of the interdisciplinary team
3. Participate in the development of the individualized plan of care
4. Address conflicts through appropriate institutional policies and procedures and other resources
5. Demonstrate professional accountability

6. Facilitate open discussion with health team members about the patient and family concerns
7. Participate in team meetings
8. Collaborates with patient and family

VII. Additional Members of the Interdisciplinary Team[1,2,4]

A. Hospice/Palliative Care Physician
1. Primary function is to consult with primary care physician and collaborate with hospice/palliative care team on management of patient's symptoms
2. Relies on the nurses who generally have more prolonged contact with the patient to provide important assessment information
3. Collaborates with all team members

B. Registered Nurse Including Advanced Practice Nurses
1. Completes the assessment of the patient and family and supervises other nursing personnel seeing the patient including the LP/VN and nursing assistant
2. Communicates assessment information and interventions
3. Collaborates with all team members
4. Advanced practice nurses may provide consultation and care management

C. Social Worker
1. Assesses strengths and resources of the patient and family system and implements interventions including emotional support
2. Provides resources to patient/families
3. Collaborates with all team members

D. Spiritual Counselor
1. Completes in-depth assessment of patient and family spiritual needs
2. Acts as liaison with community clergy when needed
3. Acts as a resource to the team on spiritual questions as well as participating in the development of the plan of care
4. Collaborates with all team members

VIII. Characteristics of a Well-Functioning Hospice and/or Palliative Care Team[5,6,10,11]

A. Members' willingness to take professional risks (e.g., share personal limitations, recognize need to get help from others)

B. Members display trust amongst each other (e.g., able to share mistakes)

C. Successes and failures are shared

D. Contributions of all members are acknowledged

E. Information shared in the team setting remains confidential and is not shared inappropriately outside of the meeting

F. There is recognition of when a team member needs assistance

G. Shared leadership activities can be a function of trust

H. Majority of members attend most meetings

I. Each member participates actively in the care planning process

J. Members treat each other with respect

K. Members seek out opinion of other members

L. Patients and families express satisfaction with the care provided by the team

M. Positive patient outcomes have traditionally been viewed as reflecting an effective team

N. Patient and family remain at the center

O. Changes in membership do not cause a major shift in outcomes

IX. Evaluation Process of the Interdisciplinary Team Functions[6-7]

   A. Monitoring performance improvement indicators

   B. Evaluating patient and family satisfaction

   C. Exit interviews when team members leave

   D. Periodic surveys of members to express concerns

CITED REFERENCES

1. Egan KA, Labyak MJ. Hospice care: a model for quality end-of-life care. In: Ferrell BR, Coyle N, eds. *Textbook of Palliative Nursing*. 2nd ed. New York, NY: Oxford University Press; 2006:13–46.

2. Center for Advancement of Palliative Care. *Designing a Palliative Care Team*. Available at: www.capc.org/building-a-hospital-based-palliative-care-program/index_html. Accessed July 6, 2009.

3. Krammer LM, Martinez J, Ring-Hurn EA, Williams MB. The nurse's role in interdisciplinary and palliative care. In: Matzo ML, Sherman DW, eds. *Palliative Nursing Care: Quality Care to the End of Life*. 3rd ed. New York, NY: Springer Publishing Company; 2010:97–106.

4. National Consensus Project. *Clinical Practice Guidelines for Quality Palliative Care*. 2nd ed. 2009. Available at: www.nationalconsensusproject.org. Accessed July 6, 2009.

5. Geriatric Interdisciplinary Team Training Curriculum. *Topic 1: Teams and Teamwork*. Available at: www.americangeriatrics.org/education/gitt/_topic.pdf. Accessed June 6, 2009.

6. Lynn J, Schuster JL, Kabcenel A. *Improving Care for the End of Life*. New York, NY: Oxford University Press; 2000.

7. Geriatric Interdisciplinary Team Training Curriculum. *Topic 3: Team Communication and Conflict Resolution*. Available at www.americangeriatrics.org/education/gitt/_topic.pdf. Accessed July 7, 2009.

8. Dahlin C, Lentz J, Sutermaster DJ. *Competencies for the Hospice and Palliative Licensed Practical/Vocational Nurse*. Dubuque, IA: Kendall Hunt Publishing; 2009.

9. Dahlin C, Lentz J, Sutermaster DJ. *Statement on the Scope and Standards of Hospice and Palliative Licensed Practical/Vocational Nursing Practice*. Dubuque, IA: Kendall Hunt Publishing; 2004.

10. Temkin-Greener H, Gross D, Kunitz SJ, Mukamel D. Measuring interdisciplinary team performance in a long-term care setting. *Medical Care*. 2004;42(5):472–481.

11. Stevenson L. The role and function of the interdisciplinary psychotherapeutic team in oncology care. In: Carroll-Johnson RM, Gorman LM, Bush NJ, eds. *Psychosocial Nursing Along the Cancer Continuum*. Pittsburgh, PA: ONS Press; 1998:277–284.

ADDITIONAL REFERENCES AND RESOURCES

Cartwright J, Kayser-Jones J. End-of-life care in assisted living facilities: perceptions of residents, families, and staffs. *Journal of Hospice and Palliative Nursing.* 2002;5(3):143–151.

Cox S, Werner B, HPNA Board of Directors. *HPNA Position Statement: Value of the Licensed Practical/ Vocational Nurse in Palliative Care.* 2008. Available at: http://www.hpna.org/DisplayPage.aspx?Title= Position Statements. Accessed December 21, 2009.

Demiris G, Washington K, Doorenbos AZ, Oliver DP, Wittenberg-Lyles E. Use of the time, interaction, and performance theory to study hospice interdisciplinary team meetings. *Journal of Hospice and Palliative Nursing.* 2008;10(6):376–381.

Egan KA, Abbott P. Interdisciplinary team training: preparing new employees for the specialty of hospice and palliative care. *Journal of Hospice and Palliative Nursing.* 2002;4(3):153–160.

Holmberg L. Communication in action between family caregivers and a palliative home care team. *Journal of Hospice and Palliative Nursing.* 2006;8(5):276–287.

Lovelady B, Sword T. Hospice care planning: an interdisciplinary roadmap. *Journal of Hospice and Palliative Nursing.* 2002;6(4):223–231.

Mazanec P, Bartel J, Buras D, Fessler P, Hudson J, Jacoby M, Montana B, Phillips M. Transdisciplinary pain management: a holistic approach. *Journal of Hospice and Palliative Nursing.* 2002;4(4):228–234.

Syme A, Bruce A. Hospice and palliative care: what unites us, what divides us? *Journal of Hospice and Palliative Nursing.* 2009;11(1):19–24.

Wittenberg-Lyles EM, Oliver DP, Demiris G, Courtney KL. Assessing the nature and process of hospice interdisciplinary team meetings. *Journal of Hospice and Palliative Nursing.* 2007;9(1):17–21.

CHAPTER III

PATTERNS OF DISEASE PROGRESSION

Beverly Paukstis, RN, MS, CHPN®, CHPA®

Adapted from: Dahlin C, Kalina K. Patterns of Disease Progression. In: Volker BG, Watson AC, eds. *Core Curriculum for the Generalist Hospice and Palliative Nurse*. Dubuque, IA: Kendall Hunt Publishing; 2005:29–61.

I. **Cancer**

    A. **Definition: Cancer is a disease of the cells. In this disease cells lose their normal controls and traits. The disease causes the cells to have unregulated growth, lack of differentiation, and provides cells with the ability to invade local tissues and then spread to other organs. This cell growth is named "tumor." The word "oncology" means the scientific study of tumors.** *Onco* **is derived from the Greek word** *onkos* **which means mass or tumor**

    B. **Cancer is the second leading cause of death in the United States**[1]

    C. **Major cancer diagnoses**

        1. Lung cancer

            a) Symptoms: cough, hemoptysis, dyspnea, pneumonia, pain in the shoulder or arm

            b) Common metastatic sites: brain, bone, liver

            c) Psychosocial issues: guilt about smoking, fear of suffocating

        2. Breast cancer

            a) Symptoms: painless mass in the breast, dimpling of skin of breast, nipple changes, one breast is different from the other, change in texture of the skin, discharge of any kind from the nipple, scaling of skin of areola or nipple

            b) Common metastatic sites: bone, liver, brain, lung

            c) Psychosocial issues: fears over losses of femininity, sexuality; perception of body as being abnormal

        3. Reproductive cancers

            a) Ovarian cancer

(1) Symptoms: increased abdominal girth, changes in bowel patterns, weight loss, vague complaints of nausea, palpable mass (in advanced stage)

(2) Common metastatic sites: lung, liver, peritoneal linings

(3) Diagnosis usually occurs late in the disease process death most likely due to the gastrointestinal complications being treated symptomatically only

(4) Genetic predisposition; tumor marker study CA-25 is recommended for prediction of disease and its presence

(5) Psychosocial issues: anger with medical system due to late diagnosis, fear of death, sexual dysfunction

b) Endometrial cancer

(1) Symptoms: changes in bowel patterns, vaginal bleeding, jaundice, ascites, dyspnea

(2) Common metastatic sites: bone, peritoneal linings

(3) Psychosocial issues: sexual dysfunction, frustration with treatment that is rarely helpful

c) Cervical cancer

(1) Symptoms: associated with metastasis to bladder because disease is not diagnosed until late in the process: dysuria, urinary retention, urinary frequency, hematuria; rectal bleeding, changes in bowel patterns

(2) Common metastatic sites: bladder, bone, genitourinary system

(3) Psychosocial issues: guilt over failure to obtain Papanicolaou test (PAP smear), guilt over sexual habits (herpes II and human papillomavirus [HPV] are precursors)

d) Testicular cancer

(1) Symptoms are not seen until late in the disease: back pain, bone pain (due to probable metastases to bone), dyspnea, seizures, headache, cough (due to probable metastasis to lung, brain)

(2) Common metastatic sites: bone, lung, liver

(3) Psychosocial issues: some clinicians and researchers have linked with high use of certain sports such as biking and baseball

(4) Despite metastasis and advanced disease, usually curable

4. Genitourinary cancers

a) Prostate cancer

(1) Symptoms initially are difficulty in urinating and hematuria progressing to painful defecation, weight loss, and worsening urinary obstruction

(2) Common metastatic sites: bone, most often the bone pain is the patient's chief complaint

b) Bladder cancer

   (1) Symptoms: hematuria, flank pain, changes in urination function (dysuria, frequency, urgency), renal failure

   (2) Common metastatic sites: genitourinary system, peritoneal linings

   (3) Psychosocial issues: potential for loss of sexuality when surgery is done; males may become impotent and in females the anterior wall of the vagina may be removed

c) Kidney cancer

   (1) Symptoms: gross hematuria, dull pain, palpable abdominal mass, fever, weight loss, dyspnea, anemia

   (2) Common metastatic sites: bone, lung, liver, brain

   (3) Psychosocial issues: guilt over cigarette smoking; there is a possible link to exposure to asbestos, cadmium and lead

5. Gastrointestinal cancers

   a) Colon, rectal, and anal cancers

      (1) Symptoms: constipation, incontinence, weight loss, sensation of rectal fullness, dull perineal or sacral pain radiating down legs, rectal bleeding

      (2) Common metastatic sites: lung, liver

      (3) Psychosocial issues: guilt over incurring what is now seen as preventable; potential for distortion of body image due to a colostomy

   b) Esophageal cancer

      (1) Symptoms: dysphasia, signs of airway obstruction, dehydration, general debilitation

      (2) Diagnosis most often occurs in advanced stages of disease, very poor prognosis

      (3) Common metastatic sites: lung, liver, adrenal glands

      (4) Psychosocial issues: disease usually grows rapidly

   c) Pancreatic cancer

      (1) Symptoms: extreme jaundice, abdominal pain, nausea, vomiting, diarrhea, feeling of fullness, bloating

      (2) Common metastatic sites: lung, liver, bowel, rectum

      (3) Psychosocial issues: depression frequently accompanies this diagnosis more than other cancer diagnoses; believed to be correlated with sugar metabolism

   d) Gastric cancer (stomach)

      (1) Symptoms: weight loss, malnutrition, weakness

      (2) Common metastatic sites: lung, liver, bowel, rectum

      (3) Psychosocial issues: in most cultures, food equals caring and often caregiver/patient stress occurs over inability to eat

e) Liver

   (1) Symptoms: bloating, weight loss, pain, bleeding, nausea, vomiting, jaundice, anorexia, itching of skin (pruritus), peripheral edema, confusion

   (2) Common metastatic sites: bone, lung

   (3) Psychosocial issues: may be associated with cirrhosis (alcoholic or nutritional) hence possible guilt over prevention; aggressive disease

6. Leukemia/malignant blood disorders

   a) Leukemia

      (1) Disorder of blood and the organs that make blood resulting in uncontrolled growth of white blood cells[2]

      (2) Symptoms: easy and frequent bruising, nose bleeds, bleeding from gums, bladder or bowel, general malaise, fever, frequent infections

      (3) Common metastatic sites: bone, bone marrow, skin, lung, brain

      (4) Psychosocial issues: remission and relapse cycles cause emotional fatigue; occurs frequently in children

   b) Multiple myeloma

      (1) Is a tumor of the plasma cells of the blood resulting in malignant masses of plasma cells spread out in the bones and tissues[2]

      (2) Symptoms: persistent and unexplained skeletal pain, recurrent bacterial infections, anemia, pathologic fractures, constipation, renal failure

      (3) Psychosocial issues: there may be long periods of remission leading to false hope of total cure

   c) Lymphoma

      (1) Is a group of malignant growths that arises in the connective tissue and the lymphatic system may be secondary to patients with AIDS

      (2) Symptom: fever, night sweats, weight loss, itching, low back pain, shortness of breath, decreased urinary output

      (3) Common metastatic sites: bone, bone marrow, skin, lung, brain

7. Melanoma

   a) Is a tumor growing in a pigmented area of skin

   b) Symptoms: a visible lesion with varieties of size, color, shape, and growth habit

   c) Common metastatic sites: bone, lung, liver, brain

   d) Psychosocial issues: guilt over possible prevention, distortion of body image secondary to tumors or surgery

8. Head and neck cancers

   a) Symptoms: pain, visible lesions and tumors in mouth, neck, head; pain, ulcerated areas

b) Common metastatic sites: skin, lung

c) Psychosocial issues: distortion of self-image, depression, social isolation, possible inability to speak due to tracheostomy

9. Brain tumor

   a) Symptoms: drowsiness, decreased attention span, mood changes, poor judgment, impaired cognitive skills, short-term memory loss, headache, vomiting, irregularities of heart rate, seizures, personality changes, malnutrition, dehydration, hiccoughs

   b) Common metastatic site: the meninges of the brain

   c) Psychosocial issues: has often been termed "lesions of the spirit" because of the ways in which mental status is attacked and altered

II. **Treatment of Cancer**

   A. **Surgery**

   1. Removal of tumor

   2. Can be curative: all tumor and a margin of surrounding tissues are removed

   3. Can be palliative: tumor is removed as much as possible to lessen pain and symptoms

   B. **Radiation Therapy**

   1. Use of radiation to remove cells in localized cancer treatment. May be curative for some cancers

   2. Use of radiation to treat tissues or organs before the disease clinically evident

   3. Promote the eradication of cells causing distressing symptoms. May be palliative for oncologic emergencies such as spinal cord compression or superior vena cava syndrome

   C. **Chemotherapy**

   1. Is the administration of medication specifically made to destroy the cells of tumors

   2. Treats cancer in 3 ways

      a) Cure: alone or with radiation and/or surgery

      b) Control: used to extend life when cure is not possible

      c) Palliate: used to relieve the distress of some symptoms and pain when neither cure nor control is possible (e.g., decrease of bowel tumor size so that stool can pass)

   3. Side effects[3]

      a) Short-term: (few days): nausea, vomiting, stomatitis, diarrhea, and anorexia

      b) Long-term: peripheral nerve damage with resulting peripheral neuropathies and pain—constipation, toxicity to kidneys, toxicity to heart, hemorrhagic bladder infection (cystitis), pulmonary fibrosis

D. **Supportive and Alternative Treatments**
   1. Blood transfusions, artificial nutrition administration (tube feedings, TPN)
   2. Complementary therapies of vitamin and herbal supplements, psychological techniques, support groups

III. **Human Immunodeficiency Virus Infection (HIV Infection)**

   A. **Definition: HIV is a group of retroviruses that invade a host cell's DNA and this results in a wide range of clinical presentations varying from no symptoms to fever, debilitation, and fatal related disorders**

   B. **Transmission requires close contact with body fluids**
      1. Contaminated blood products
      2. Sexual contact: rectal, vaginal
      3. Organ transplant and insemination from infected donors
      4. Prenatal and perinatal exposure for newborns (pregnancy, childbirth, breastfeeding)
      5. Occupational injuries such as needle sticks, sharps sticks. Sharing of contaminated needles by IV drug users

   C. **Can be managed with retroviral drugs**

   D. **Cluster of symptoms: malaise, fatigue, weight loss, intermittent fever, chronic diarrhea, lymphadenopathy**

IV. **Acquired Immunodeficiency Syndrome (AIDS)**

   A. **Definition: infection with HIV that leads to the development of opportunistic infections and/or certain secondary cancers such as Kaposi's sarcoma and non-Hodgkin's lymphoma, and neurological dysfunction**

   B. **Symptoms**
      1. Neurologic: seizures, focal motor sensory or gait disturbances, headache, lethargy
      2. Infections: pneumonia, meningitis, encephalitis, thrush

   C. **Psychosocial Issues: social isolation, depression, fear of death, guilt over possible prevention, anger. Issues related to disenfranchisement**

   D. **Neither HIV nor AIDS can be cured. HIV can be maintained and held in check with retroviral medications. AIDS requires treatment of symptoms; it cannot be controlled or held in check**

E. **AIDS occurs when people cannot tolerate or do not take retroviral medications for HIV infection**

F. **Special grief issues in AIDS bereavement care**
   1. These issues surface for the patient in the category of anticipatory grief
      a) Stigma of AIDS and HIV leads to social isolation
      b) Stigma of substance abuse
      c) Guilt over behaviors that may be causes
   2. These issues may surface for members of the family and friends
      a) Homophobia
      b) Multiple losses
      c) Disenfranchised grief

V. **Neurological Conditions**

   A. **Causes**
      1. Injury (internal)
         a) Cerebrovascular accident (CVA): 3rd leading cause of deaths in USA, resulting in death of brain cells due to clots (embolism) in a blood vessel, rupture in a vessel or of an aneurysm, or due to the presence of plaque in the cerebral blood vessels, damage depends on location and size
      2. Injury (external)
         a) Trauma to skull
         b) Intracranial or subdural bleeding and prolonged pressure within the brain and skull leads to damages similar to CVA
      3. Degenerative diseases
         a) Amyotrophic lateral sclerosis (ALS): a motor neuron disease in the cerebral cortex, the brainstem, the spinal cord. Results in progressive weakness and atrophy of muscles. Usually there is no change in mentation
         b) Dementia: Alzheimer's disease or other type: an irreversible and progressive dementia characterized by mentation deterioration, disorganization of personality, results in total inability to execute any daily living tasks including eating
         c) Parkinson's disease: idiopathic, slowly progressing degenerative disorder of the CNS characterized by slow movements, muscle rigidity, resting tremor, and postural instability

   B. **Treatment**
      1. Medications to relieve the symptoms, such as steroids for injuries to the brain
      2. ALS and Alzheimer's disease have trials of drugs in process

3. Functional care focuses on re-establishing or maintaining ADLs, providing appropriate nutrition, preventing complications related to being immobile

4. Psychosocial support to patient and to family

C. **Consideration in Advanced Disease**

1. Injury: permanent neurological damage predisposes to complications: dysphasia, incontinence, infections. Death is usually related to subsequent CVAs or major infection

2. Degenerative diseases: progressive weakness, dysphasia, respiratory diminishment, infections and seizures as well as immobility all contribute to the dying process

VI. **Cardiac Conditions**

A. **This category includes diseases of the heart which cause damage to the heart muscle through various mechanisms that result in loss of oxygen to the heart or decreased cardiac output**

B. **Causes**

1. Half of the cases are idiopathic (unknown cause)

2. The rest can be the result of chronic high alcohol intake, inherited tendencies, metabolic and endocrine diseases, infection, and coronary artery disease

C. **Treatment**

1. Surgical: heart transplant, angioplasty, bypass surgery

2. Pharmacologic: diuretics, nitrates, morphine, calcium channel blockers, beta blockers, ACE inhibitors, vasodilators, glycosides

3. Cardiac rehab, diet changes, stress management

D. **Advanced Disease**

1. Congestive heart failure (CHF): failure of the heart to be able to function properly due to an accumulation of situations that prevent adequate performance. These are conditions that no longer or never could respond to treatment modalities

2. Symptoms of congestive heart failure: anxiety, restlessness, dyspnea, tachycardia, palpitations, lung wheezes, fatigue, cyanosis or pallor, dependent peripheral edema, weight gain, cough, hemoptysis

3. Psychosocial issue: inability to resolve impending death due to success of previous rescue efforts through drugs or CPR/ventilator

VII. **Pulmonary Diseases**

A. **Lung Diseases are Either Obstructive or Restrictive**

1. Obstructive (chronic obstructive pulmonary disease—COPD): small airways have chronic spasms caused by disease, tobacco, toxins

a) Emphysema: damage to the airways due to elastin breakdown which causes a decreased ability of alveolar to expel air. Dyspnea is the result of air trapped in the aveoli.[4] Symptoms

   (1) Patient has muscle wasting progressive external dyspnea

   (2) Accessory muscles are used for breathing

   (3) Chest is "barrel" in appearance, patient cannot cough well, breath sounds are weak

b) Chronic bronchitis: increased secretion of thick 'sticky' mucous that increases risk of pulmonary infections. Chronic cough is the result of mucous and is difficult to clear due to damaged cilia and thickened inflamed bronchial walls.[4] Symptoms

   (1) Patient is overweight

   (2) Cyanosis is present

   (3) Breath is wheezing

2. Restrictive: loss of lung tissues which causes limited lung expansion due to other diseases such as cancer, fibrosis, and myasthenia gravis

B. Treatment

1. For COPD: pharmacologic (bronchodilators, corticosteroids, xanthenes, anticholinergics), oxygen

2. For restricted lung disease: pharmacologic (e.g., corticosteroids, nebulizers/IPPB), oxygen

C. Advanced Disease

1. Both types of lung disease eventually result in lung failure

2. Management of symptoms is focused on comfort

   a) Medication regimens that are supplemented by anti-anxiety agents and morphine

   b) Mechanisms and techniques that promote calm: massage, imaging, hypnosis, relaxation, purse lip breathing

D. Psychosocial Issues: guilt over lifestyles that may have caused disease and fear of suffocation

VIII. Kidney Diseases

A. The inability of kidneys to function is called "renal failure." The causes include toxins, some medications, tumors, infections, diabetes, hypertension, collagen vascular diseases such as lupus or scleroderma

B. Treatment

1. Dialysis: peritoneal or hemodialysis is useful in short-term renal failure when the kidneys are expected to resume function; may also be used long-term when there is no expectation of return of kidney function

2. Surgery: debulking of tumors, insertion of nephrostomy tubes

3. Pharmacologic: diuretics, dietary management, treatment of underlying causes such as antihypertensives

4. Nutrition: focuses on low sodium, low protein, low potassium foods

C. **Advanced Disease**

1. Fluid and electrolyte imbalance, anemia, uremia

2. Treatment is focused on comfort through medication

3. Psychosocial issues: most compelling is the decision to continue or stop dialysis

IX. **General Debility**

A. **Debility, unspecified, is now a diagnostic category for elderly and debilitated persons with functional disabilities and progressive multiple organ failure who do not meet the criteria specific for other terminal diseases. This diagnosis takes the place of the pediatric "failure to thrive," which was used for this condition**

B. **Performance Scales**

1. Karnofsky Performance Scale (KPS)[5]

    a) 0 to 100 scale used to rate a patient's ability to do their own activities of daily living

    b) The higher the rating the less care needed

2. EGOC Performance Status[6]

    a) 0 to 5 scale used to assess how a patient's disease is affecting their ability to do activities of daily living

    b) The lower the rating, the less restrictions

3. Palliative Performance Scale (PPSv2)[7]

    a) 0% to 100% scale of five areas to communicate a patient's current level of functioning. The areas are ambulation, activity and evidence of disease, self-care, intake and conscious level

    b) The higher the score, the more independent

C. **Symptoms**

1. Severe deficits in ADLs

2. Poor performance scale rating

3. Signs and symptoms of multiple organ failure

4. Progressive physical deterioration

D. **Treatment**
1. Symptom management
2. Appropriate nutrition
3. Prevention of complications

E. **Advanced disease treatment is focused on comfort through medications and provision of personal care**

X. **Endocrine Diseases**

A. **Diabetes mellitus (DM): a group of disorders distinguished by chronic hyperglycemia, difficulties of carbohydrate, fat, and protein metabolism[8]; leading cause of kidney failure. There are 3 types**
1. Type 1: almost complete loss of insulin production by the B-cells of the islet of Langerhans in the pancreas. Commonly diagnosed in children. Initial symptoms include weight loss and increased thirst, hunger and urination from the lack of insulin to transport glucose into the cells. Without glucose entering the cells, the body will lose weight prompting feelings of polyphagia. The excess glucose is excreted by the kidneys which takes a large amount of water with it resulting in polyuria. After the loss of the water the body wants to drink more fluids resulting in polydipsia. Treatment includes insulin injections, a diet tailored to meet the individual's needs usually with a calorie restriction and close monitoring of blood glucose level[8]
2. Type 2: cells become resistant to insulin, which results in high levels of insulin in the blood that cannot transport glucose into the cells. Seen mostly in adults. Symptoms are not always specific but can include being overweight, lipid disturbances, and hypertension. Treatment can include weight control, diet with reduced calories, medications, and close monitoring of blood glucose levels. There are multiple antidiabetic medications that can increase insulin secretion, decrease glucose production and aid cells in accepting the insulin[8]
3. Other causes of hyperglycemia: gestational diabetes, impaired glucose tolerance as well as pancreatic injury, infection, corticosteroid use, and cancer. These causes may result in diabetes mellitus[8]

B. **Treatment is directed toward maintaining control of blood sugar through insulin, oral antidiabetic drugs, diet, blood sugar monitoring, and patient teaching**

C. **Advanced disease**
1. Failure to adhere to control regimen can result in death at any time
2. Complications of DM; peripheral vascular disease, coronary artery disease, diabetic neuropathy, kidney failure, infections, impaired wound healing

D. **Treatment focuses on comfort through the use of medications**

E. **Psychosocial issues: anger directed toward patient by family for the perceived failure to adhere to a control regimen**

CITED REFERENCES

1. Centers for Disease Control and Prevention, National Center for Health Statistics. *National Vital Statistics Report*. 2009. Available at: www.cdc.gov/nchs/data/nvsr/nvsr57/nvsr57_14.pdf. Accessed February 2, 2010.

2. Mansen TJ, McCance KL. Alterations in leukocyte, lymphoid and hemostatic function. In: McCance KL, Huether SE, eds. *Pathophysiology: The Biologic Basis for Disease in Adults and Children*. 4th ed. St. Louis, MO: Mosby; 2002:865–899.

3. Yarbo CH, Frogge MH, Goodman M, eds. *Cancer Nursing: Principles and Practice*. 6th ed. Boston, MA: Jones and Bartlett Publishers; 2005.

4. Brashers VL. Alterations in pulmonary function. In: McCance KL, Huether SE, eds. *Pathophysiology: The Biologic Basis for Disease in Adults and Children*. 4th ed. St. Louis, MO: Mosby; 2002:1105–1144.

5. *Karnofsky Performance Scale Index*. Available at: www.hospicepatients.org/karnofsky.html. Accessed February 3, 2010.

6. Eastern Cooperative Oncology Group. *ECOG Performance Status*. 2006. Available at: www.ecog.org/general/perf_stat.html. Accessed February 3, 2010.

7. Victoria Hospice Society. *Palliative Performance Scale (PPSv2)*. 2001. Available at: palliative.info/resource_material/PPSv2.pdf. Accessed February 3, 2010.

8. Jones RE, Huether SE. Alterations in hormonal regulation. In: McCance KL, Huether SE, eds. *Pathophysiology: The Biologic Basis for Disease in Adults and Children*. 4th ed. St. Louis, MO: Mosby; 2002:624–669.

Additional References and Resources

Buck HG, McMillan SC. The unmet spiritual needs of caregivers of patients with advanced cancer. *Journal of Hospice and Palliative Nursing.* 2008;10(2):91–99.

Cooper DH, Krainik AJ, Lubner SJ, et al. *The Washington Manual of Medical Therapeutics.* 2nd ed. St. Louis, MO: Washington University School of Medicine; 2007.

Ferrell BR, Coyle N, eds. *Textbook of Palliative Nursing.* 3rd ed. New York, NY: Oxford University Press; 2010.

Hanks G, Cherny NI, Christakis NA, Fallon M, Kaasa S, Portenoy RK, eds. *Oxford Textbook of Palliative Medicine.* 4th ed. New York, NY: Oxford University Press; 2009.

Hayajneh FA, Al-Hussami M. Predictors of quality of life among women living with human immunodeficiency virus/AIDS. *Journal of Hospice and Palliative Nursing.* 2009;11(5):255–261.

Hemani S, Letizia M. Providing palliative care in end-stage heart failure. *Journal of Hospice and Palliative Nursing.* 2008;10(2):100–105.

Houseman G. Symptom management of the patient with amyotrophic lateral sclerosis: a guide for hospice nurses. *Journal of Hospice and Palliative Nursing.* 2008;10(4):207–213.

Langford R, Thompson J, eds. *Mosby's Handbook of Diseases.* 3rd ed. St. Louis, MO: Mosby; 2005.

Mazanec P, Daly BJ, Pitorak EF, et al. A new model of palliative care for oncology patients with advanced disease. *Journal of Hospice and Palliative Nursing.* 2009;11(6):324–331.

Meixner E. Palliative care and the acute stroke patient. *Journal of Hospice and Palliative Nursing.* 2009;11(6):310.

Morgan BD, Kochan KA. I'll always want more: complex issues in HIV palliative care. *Journal of Hospice and Palliative Nursing.* 2008;10(5):265–271.

CHAPTER IV

PAIN MANAGEMENT

Tami Borneman, RN, PHN, MSN, CNS, FPCN
Lynda Gruenwald-Schmitz, RN, MSN, CHPN®

Adapted from: Berry PH, Paice JA. Patient care: pain management. In: Volker BG, Watson AC, eds. *Core Curriculum for the Generalist Hospice and Palliative Nurse*. Dubuque, IA: Kendall Hunt Publishing; 2002:63–87.

I. **Introduction**

   A. **Overview**

      1. Prevalence

         a) Pain is experienced by 70–90% of patients with advanced disease, 40–50% of patients experience moderate pain, and 25–30% have severe pain

         b) Pain scores (on a 0–10 scale) greater than or equal to "5" greatly impact on quality of life

      2. It is estimated that almost all patients (85–90%) could be free of pain and 98–99% pain controlled using the knowledge and tools currently available; the remaining 1–2% of patients at end of life can be offered palliative sedation (defined as providing relief of refractory and intolerable symptoms with the use of sedatives at the end of life) in addition to analgesics

         a) This practice is within the realm of good supportive palliative care and is <u>not</u> euthanasia. The goal of sedation is to relieve distress from unrelenting physical, psychological or spiritual symptoms

         b) This was formerly referred to as *terminal sedation*, however this term led to confusion, suggesting assisted suicide, and the preferred terminology is palliative sedation

   B. **Barriers to Both the Assessment and the Treatment of Pain**

      1. Barriers from the patient and family perspective

         a) *Good* patients do not complain

         b) Pain is inevitable with aging

         c) Strong medicine only comes in injectable form

d) Bearing the pain is better than bearing the side effects of pain medicine

e) Addiction to pain medicine is common

f) Strong pain medicine should only be used for very severe pain

g) Morphine is a *last ditch drug* used only when one is imminently dying

h) Fear of disease getting worse

2. Barriers from the nurse and physician perspective

   a) The patient's self report of pain is not believed: healthcare professionals are the best judge of pain

   b) In the hospital setting, pain is often not seen as important as other indicators

   c) Only opioids are effective in severe pain

   d) Opioids cause respiratory depression

   e) Double effect: an ethical principle that permits an action, intended to have a good effect, when there is a risk of also causing a harmful effect, ONLY when the intention was to produce the good effect

      (1) Double effect, as a principle guiding care, is complex, but nonetheless erroneously applied to end-of-life care, especially pain and symptom management

      (2) Adequately controlling symptoms at end of life is not known to shorten life

      (3) An analysis of the potential benefits of a therapy weighed against the possible risks should be conducted when considering any therapy

   f) The confusion over addiction/tolerance/physical dependence (see below)

   g) General lack of education relating to pain assessment, treatment, and pharmacology in basic and graduate education programs

      (1) There are still physicians and nurses who believe that morphine kills patients

      (2) There is a lack of knowledge regarding the treatment of chronic versus acute pain

3. Other barriers that impact on reporting pain and using analgesics

   a) Anti-drug, "opio-phobic" culture—"Just say 'no' to drugs"

   b) Restrictions that vary by state, including triplicate prescription laws or other programs that monitor provider prescribing patterns, lack of laws facilitating pain management in end stage illness, including partial filling of scheduled medications (fractioning)

C. **Important Definitions**

1. Pain: pain is whatever the experiencing person says it is, existing whenever he/she says it does.[1] History is 80% of the diagnosis. The patient's subjective report of pain is even more important to an accurate diagnosis, as there are no physical exam techniques or diagnostic tests to confirm pain history—***the patient's report must be accepted!***

2. Addiction: overwhelming involvement with obtaining and using a drug for its psychic benefits; not for medical reason; behavior is compulsive and subject to relapse; *quality of life is not improved or enhanced; use continues despite harm*

3. Tolerance: after repeated administration of an opioid, a given dosage begins to lose its effectiveness; first in duration of action; second in overall effectiveness. Dose should be gradually titrated upward to maintain the effectiveness of the opioid

4. Analgesic ceiling: a dose beyond which additional analgesic effect is not obtained

5. Physical dependence: after repeated administration of an opioid, withdrawal symptoms occur when the drug is not taken

   a) Signs and symptoms of abstinence syndrome (withdrawal) include anxiety, irritability, lacrimation, rhinorrhea, sweating, nausea, vomiting, cramps, insomnia, and (rarely) multifocal myoclonus

   b) Appearance of abstinence syndrome is a function of the elimination half-life of the opioid; for example, abstinence symptoms appear between 6–12 hours and peak between 24–72 hours following the last dose of a medication with a short half-life (morphine is an example)

   c) Conversely, with medications with a longer half-life, the appearance of abstinence symptoms are delayed, for example, with methadone, as much as 36 to 48 hours

6. Opioid "pseudo-addiction": an iatrogenic syndrome in which patients develop certain behavioral characteristics of psychological dependence as a consequence of inadequate pain treatment[2,3]

7. Palliative care: active total treatment and care of patients whose disease is not responsive to curative treatment. Control of pain, other symptoms, and of psychological, social, and spiritual problems is paramount. The goal of palliative care is achievement of the best possible quality of life for patients and their families. Many aspects of palliative care are also applicable earlier in the course of the illness, in conjunction with anticancer treatment. Palliative care encompasses several different settings where terminal patients receive their care including hospice and home health settings, long-term care facilities and acute care hospitals. Palliative care utilizes a team approach[4]

II. **Assessment of Pain: effectiveness of pain management is directly related to assessment**

   A. **Types of Pain**

   1. Acute pain: usually clear cause; meaningful; perceived as reversible; observable signs (i.e., increased pulse rate and blood pressure; nonverbal signs and symptoms, such as facial expressions, tense muscles)

      a) Examples: myocardial infarction, acute appendicitis

   2. Chronic or persistent: often not a clear cause; does not fulfill a useful purpose; perceived as irreversible; cyclical (aching—agony); decreased social interaction, insomnia, depressed effect; few observable or behavioral signs

      a) Examples: cancer pain, chronic back pain

3. Nociceptive pain (or somatic and visceral pain) arises from direct stimulation of the afferent nerves due to tumor infiltration, of skin, soft tissue, or viscera

    a) Somatic pain: well-localized; often described as deep, dull ache; musculoskeletal in nature

        (1) Examples: bone metastasis, inflammation of soft tissue, tumor invasion of soft tissue

        (2) Can be controlled with conventional analgesics (including NSAIDs if mild, and opioids, if moderate to severe), and in some cases, radiation therapy

    b) Visceral pain: poorly localized; cramping, deep ache, pressure, often referred to distant dermatome sites

        (1) Examples: bowel obstruction, cholecystitis; metastatic tumors in the lung

        (2) Can be controlled with conventional analgesics, and in some cases, antineoplastic treatments

4. Neuropathic pain results from actual injury to nerves rather than stimulation of nerve endings (refer to Table 1 for Pain Terms Associated with Neuropathic Pain States)

    a) Characteristics: sharp, burning, shooting, shock-like, sometimes associated with acyclovir and dysesthesias

    b) Examples: spinal nerve root compression, tumor invasion of nerves, post-herpetic neuralgia, surgical interruption of nerves, central pain syndromes occurring after stroke

    c) Response to conventional analgesics often poor (although this is controversial); but antidepressants (e.g., nortriptyline), anticonvulsants (e.g., gabapentin, carbamazepine), corticosteroids, and non-drug therapies may be beneficial as adjuvant analgesics to the opioids or in some cases as the primary analgesic. Adjuvant analgesics are medications that have a primary indication other than pain; however they contain analgesic properties of various pain conditions. Adjuvant medications can be used as an add-on to an existing opioid regimen or as a primary therapy for pain where good results are likely to occur[5]

5. Mixed nociceptive and neuropathic pain syndrome

    a) Common in life-threatening illnesses

    b) Thorough assessment is indicated

        (1) Pharmacological therapy is based upon these different pain syndromes

        (2) Occur concomitantly so patients may require agents from more than one category of analgesics (e.g., non-opioids, opioids, and adjuvants)

6. Referred pain is usually a visceral pain referred to skin, bone, and muscle, often distant from the site of origin

    a) Pain from tumor involvement of the pancreas, lower esophagus, stomach, or retroperitoneal area may be referred to the back

b) Gallbladder or liver disease may produce referred pain in the back or right shoulder (suprascapular)

c) Rectosigmoid involvement may result in pain to sacrum or rectal area

B. Assessment Parameters

1. Site: have patient point on self or diagram, identify and assess all sites as well as sites of radiation; remember, also, the patient may have more than one site of pain; in that case, it would be helpful to number pains to organize assessment, interventions, and evaluations

2. Character: use the patient's <u>own</u> words; a careful description will lead to the diagnosis of pain type, and therefore use of appropriate adjuvant analgesics (i.e., sharp, shooting describes neuropathic pain syndromes); refer to the section, "Types of Pain," for additional, in depth descriptions

3. Onset: when did it start? Did (or does) a specific event trigger the pain?

   a) Carefully distinguish between new and pre-existing pain (i.e., arthritis, chronic low back pain syndromes, etc.)

   b) Also assess for breakthrough pain

   (1) Transient flares of pain in patients with chronic pain syndromes are referred to as breakthrough pain

   (2) Breakthrough pain can be incidental (e.g., associated with movement), idiopathic (i.e., the cause is not known), or can occur as end-of-dose failure (e.g., the pain recurs prior to the next dose of pain medication)

4. Duration and frequency: how long has the pain persisted? Is it constant or does it come and go (intermittent)?

5. Intensity: *Important note: ratings of pain intensity are the most important piece of pain assessment data to obtain if time is short; pain intensity directly correlates with interference with the patient's quality of life*

   a) Commonly defined on a scale, most frequently 0–10, intensity rating method must be adapted to patient. Record pain intensity "now," at its "worst," at its "least" and on an average. Pain rating scales for cognitively impaired or nonverbal patients are available, but caregivers (be they family or staff in a care facility) can often give valuable information to add to the pain assessment

   b) A change in the patient's behavior, however, is considered the "gold standard"

   c) Indicators of the presence of pain in patients who are unable to respond include the furrowed brow and grimacing

   d) Relief of the furrowing is often seen when pain is relieved; likewise, response to treatment can be considered part of the assessment

   e) Several different pain assessment tools exist, but the basic information is similar. See below for sample tools

Figure 1: Numerical Rating Scale (NRS)

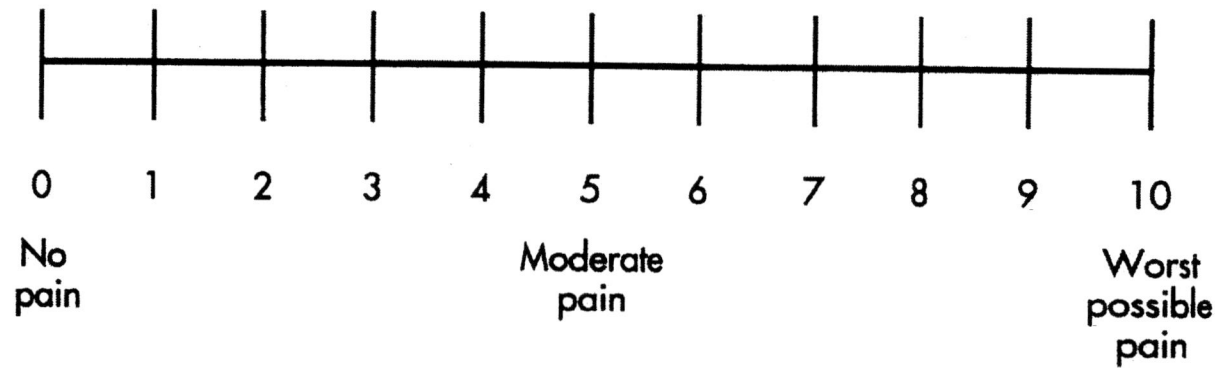

May be duplicated for use in clinical practice. As appears in: McCaffery M, Pasero C. *Pain: Clinical Manual*. St. Louis: MO: Mosby; 1999:67.

Figure 2: Wong-Baker Faces Pain Rating Scale

Modified from: Wong DL. *Whaley and Wong's Essentials of Pediatric Nursing*. 5th ed. St. Louis, MO: Mosby; 1997: 1215–1216.

6. Exacerbating factors: what times, activities, or other circumstances make the pain worse?

7. Associated symptoms: what other symptoms occur before, with or after the pain?

8. Alleviating factors: what makes the pain better? What treatments (including non-pharmacologic interventions) have been successful in the past and what unsuccessful? Include a thorough medication history

9. Medication history: what medications have been ordered? What medications is the patient currently taking? If there is a disparity, examine the underlying reasons (e.g., cost, adverse effects, and fears of addiction or tolerance). What medications worked in the past for unrelated pain episodes? What are the patient and family/caregivers' beliefs about opioids?

10. Impact on quality of life: what does the pain mean to the patient and family? How has this pain affected them and their quality of life? Does it keep the patient from doing things he/she wants to do? How much does the patient and the family know about pain? Do they have the expectation that it can be relieved? Are there emotional or spiritual components to the pain? Does unrelieved pain lead to increased fear or anxiety, or to fears that death is imminent?

11. Physical examination: observe the site of the pain, and validate with the patient the pain's location; note skin color, warmth, irritation, integrity and any other unusual findings; utilize other physical assessment techniques, for example, percussion and auscultation, as appropriate; be mindful that persons with chronic or persistent pain often have no changes in vital signs or facial expression

C. Etiology of Pain

1. Cancer pain syndromes

    a) Pain associated with direct tumor involvement

    (1) Direct tumor involvement accounts for approximately 78% of pain problems among cancer inpatients and 62% among cancer outpatients

    (2) Examples include metastatic bone disease, nerve compression or infiltration, hollow viscus involvement, among others

    b) Pain associated with cancer therapy

    (1) Cancer therapy accounts for approximately 19% of pain problems among cancer inpatients and 25% among cancer outpatients

    (2) Examples include any pain that occurs in the course of or as a result of surgery, chemotherapy or radiation therapy (specific examples are mucositis, peripheral neuropathy, phantom pain syndromes, extravasation of vesicant chemotherapy)

    c) Pain unrelated to cancer or cancer therapy

    (1) Incident pain accounts for approximately 3% of pain problems among cancer inpatients and 10% of pain problems among cancer outpatients

    (2) Examples include arthritis, osteoporosis, migraine headache, low back pain, fibromyalgia, or any other pain syndromes present among the general population

    (3) Incident pain can also refer to pain that is the result of activity or no movement at all. Breakthrough pain is a type of incident pain

2. Pain syndromes common in the terminal phase of other medical conditions

    a) HIV infection and AIDS

    (1) Statistics on the prevalence of pain in AIDS range from 30 to 97%, with an estimate of 50% relating directly to the HIV infection and 30% to the therapy for AIDS

    (2) HIV pain is often categorized in a manner similar to cancer: pain associated with the virus (e.g., direct involvement of the virus in the sensory neurons that transmit pain), pain associated with the treatment (e.g., neuropathy due to antiretroviral drugs) or pain unrelated to HIV or its treatment (e.g., musculoskeletal pains after exercise)

    (3) Examples of HIV/AIDS related pain include neuropathies (specifically peripheral neuropathy, acute and chronic polyneuropathy, symmetric distal sensory neuropathy, brachial plexopathy, herpetic neuralgia, cranial neuropathy, and headaches from acute and chronic meningitis), central pain from cerebral abscesses, esophagitis and abdominal pain from infectious gastrointestinal disease, chest pain from pneumocystis pneumonia, and generalized myalgias

b) Sickle cell disease

   (1) Three or more vascular occlusive episodes are a poor prognostic sign (less than 50% of those patients live beyond age 40). Hydroxyurea may decrease frequency of vasoocclusive crises

   (2) Pain is severe and acute; focal (bone, joint and muscle) and visceral pain from ischemia and infarction

   (3) There are multiple myths and mistaken beliefs about sickle cell disease and sickle cell pain on the part of patients, their families, and the healthcare professions

   (4) Factors related to race, ethnic, and class stereotyping in our culture further complicate this issue and serve as additional impediments to the control of pain in sickle cell disease[6]

c) Multiple sclerosis (MS)

   (1) Pain is an issue in 55 to 82% of persons with MS

      i. Neurological (paroxysmal trigeminal neuralgia, optic neuritis and periorbital pain, extremity pain, including dysesthesia, allodynia, and painful electric-shock sensations)

      ii. Musculoskeletal (low back pain and extremity pain) in nature (refer to Table 1 for Pain Terms Associated with Neuropathic Pain States)

d) Cerebral vascular disease

   (1) Post-stroke pain is a problem in 1–2% of patients

      i. Often delayed for several years after the stroke; accompanied by decreased temperature sensation; may be superficial or deep; often severe in intensity and accompanied by hyperalgesia and allodynia; may be elicited by emotional episodes and movement

      ii. Another common post-stroke pain syndrome is mechanical shoulder pain unrelated to the central injury

e) Spinal cord injury: central pain may occur from an injury at any level of the spinal cord

D. Factors that may influence the experience of pain: pain is experienced by the patient *and* family in keeping with the model of "total pain" and includes physical, psychological, social, and spiritual effects; when adequate assessment and management of controllable symptoms precede psychological, social and spiritual assessment and intervention, overall outcomes often improve (remember the lesson in Maslow's Hierarchy of Needs); common effects of pain include

1. Physical effects: decreased functional ability, including ability to walk and perform other basic ADLs, decreased strength and endurance, nausea, anorexia, insomnia, and impaired immune response

2. Psychosocial effects: alteration in social and close relationships, isolation, inability to work; loss of self-esteem, self-worth; increased caregiver burden, further disruption of important social supports for both patient and family

3. Emotional effects: diminished leisure, increased fear and anxiety, depression, hopelessness, despair, loss of control; if pain uncontrolled, consideration of suicide or physician assisted suicide

4. Spiritual issues: increased suffering, re-evaluation and perhaps doubt regarding past religious foundations and beliefs; questioning the meaning of suffering

5. Financial effects: inability to work and earn income, loss of caregiver income, issues of workplace discrimination, and having to apply for governmental assistance leading to decreased income and loss of health insurance coverage

6. Cultural issues: ethnic minority, female, and elderly persons often receive less than optimal pain management in all settings[7-9]

    a) Consider the patient's family of origin, their manner of expressing pain, and how suffering is valued

    b) Perceptions of pain, end of life, afterlife, bereavement and other aspects of palliative care vary widely by ethnicity and within ethnicities

    c) Be careful of "stereotyping," and do everything possible to learn about the patient and family's unique situation

    d) Specific aspects of culture to assess when caring for patients in pain include ethnic identity, gender, age, differing abilities, sexual orientation, religion and spirituality, financial status, place of residency, employment, and educational level

III. Pharmacologic Intervention[a]

A. Types of Pharmacologic Interventions

1. Drug actions and side effects

    a) Aspirin-like drugs (NSAIDs: salicylates, and non-salicylates)

       (1) Actions: analgesic, antipyretic, anti-inflammatory, antithrombotic

       (2) Adverse effects

           i. Gastrointestinal distress; no relation between symptoms and seriousness of gastrointestinal effects; concomitant administration of misoprostol (Cytotec®) or a proton pump inhibitor (e.g., omeprazole [Prilosec®]) can prevent gastropathy

           ii. Renal insufficiency: elderly and dehydrated are at increased risk

           iii. Inhibiting of platelet aggregation

           iv. Hypersensitivity reactions (not allergic reactions); symptoms include urticaria, bronchospasm, severe rhinitis, and shock

               1. Adverse effects are often labeled by patients/caregivers as *allergies* (e.g., nausea and vomiting)

               2. These are not absolute contraindications to using the drug

           v. CNS effects: dizziness, tinnitus, decreased hearing, headache

---

[a]Thanks to June L. Dahl, PhD, Professor of Pharmacology at the University of Wisconsin-Madison Medical School for her assistance with this section.

(3) Dose escalation is limited by analgesic ceiling

b) Acetaminophen

(1) Actions: analgesic, antipyretic, *not anti-inflammatory*

(2) Adverse effects: far fewer than with NSAIDs; hepatotoxic in large doses; ceiling is 4 grams a day, lower in alcoholic patients, AIDS patients, patients with liver metastasis or those with active liver disease. Dose escalation is limited by analgesic ceiling—consider quantity of acetaminophen in combination medications (refer to Table 2)

c) Opioid medications

(1) Pure agonists (morphine is prototype, others include fentanyl, hydrocodone, hydromorphone, methadone, oxycodone)

(2) Mixed agonist-antagonists: pentazocine (Talwin®), butorphanol (Stadol®), nalbuphine (Nubain®); *not recommended for the treatment of cancer pain due to analgesic ceiling, psychotomimetic effect, precipitation of withdrawal when given to patients on opioids*

(3) Action: bind to receptors in the brain, spinal cord and in periphery

(4) Side effects of opioids

　i. Tolerance develops in days to weeks[2,3] to the sedative, emetic and respiratory depressant effects of opioids; however it does not develop to constipation

　ii. Sedation, sometimes, but rarely confusion

　iii. Dizziness, dysphoria

　iv. Nausea

　v. Constipation: tolerance <u>does</u> <u>not</u> develop—*must be prevented and treated aggressively*

　vi. Itching and urticaria

　vii. Respiratory depression

　　1. Feared and misunderstood

　　2. Clinically significant respiratory depression is extremely rare when patients in severe pain receive opioids, especially in patients who are currently receiving opioids and when doses are titrated upward in appropriate steps; there are not good data to support the prevalence of respiratory depression due to opioids, however, there is general agreement that patients who are at risk are those who are opioid naïve and concomitantly taking other sedating drugs

　　3. Respiratory rate alone is not an indicator of respiratory depression; some patients may have a respiratory rate of 7, while alert and well perfused; other factors that must be considered are the level of sedation, the depth of respiration, and the adequacy of perfusion of oxygen in the tissues as determined by examining nail beds for changes in color, or obtaining an oxygen saturation level or pulse oximetry

(5) Some other drug adverse effects include

    i. Meperidine (Demerol®)

        1. Converted to a long-lived excitatory metabolite (normeperidine) causing shaky feelings, tremors/twitches, and myoclonus/grand mal seizures; should not be used in cancer pain management, can cause hallucinations and is contraindicated for elders

        2. Poor oral bioavailability

        3. Not recommended for use in palliative care

    ii. Propoxyphene, the opioid in Darvon® and Darvocet®

        1. Ineffective analgesic

        2. Long-lived metabolite toxic to the central nervous system and cardiovascular system

        3. Combined with a large amount of acetaminophen. Therefore, it is not recommended for long-term use or use in the elderly. No more than 4 grams of acetaminophen should be given in 24 hours due to its toxic effect on the liver

    iii. Morphine

        1. Active metabolites (morphine 3-glucuronide[M3G], morphine 6-glucuronide[M6G]), excreted by the kidneys will be retained by elderly patients and by those with diminished renal function; has strong analgesic and respiratory depressant properties; M3G may produce central nervous system hyper-excitability and possibly myoclonus, while elevated M6G levels appear to cause sedation

        2. Small amounts of hydration (IV fluids at 30–50cc/hr) help to clear it through the kidneys

        3. Hydromorphone may be a safer choice for the elderly or those with diminished renal function

    iv. Methadone

        1. Can have an effect on heart rhythms; EKG may need to be checked before methadone is started

(6) Most opioids do not have a ceiling dose: so able to titrate to effect. Check with your pharmacist for those that have a ceiling dose

    i. All mixed agonist/antagonists do have dosage ceilings and thus cannot be titrated to effect

    ii. Opioids that are administered in combination with another medication such as acetaminophen or aspirin, do have dose limitations due to the acetaminophen or aspirin

    iii. Some long-acting opioids have a ceiling limit due to the other ingredients in the pill

(7) Delivery routes

    i. Oral: most preferred for comfort, convenience, and cost effectiveness; many forms available, immediate release tablets, sustained release tablets, liquids; Oralet® (fentanyl) is available as well. Sublingual is same as oral route

    ii. Rectal: useful for patients who are NPO or have nausea and vomiting; contraindicated with anal lesions, diarrhea, constipation, or leukopenia; varying comfort levels with family caregivers and some cultures

    iii. Subcutaneous or intravenous infusion: rarely required, but useful for pain requiring rapid titration of medication; while subcutaneous infusion is useful in most cases, impaired circulation or the presence of fibrosis can compromise absorption; used extensively at home for patients who are obstructed or who can no longer swallow and have severe pain. Can be managed within home setting; especially useful if parenteral route required and reliable or intravenous access not possible. Expense of home parenteral infusions to hospice programs are a barrier to use

    iv. Intramuscular injections should be avoided, injections are painful, unnecessary and absorption is not reliable

    v. Transmucosal: easily accessible route, provides rapid onset of action and is much faster if used with lipophilic drugs such as fentanyl

    vi. Transdermal (e.g., fentanyl) for patients with stable pain (not good for rapid titration of medication); reservoir in subcutaneous tissue, delayed onset of action (12–24 hours), so patient must have an immediate release medication during the first several hours after the fentanyl patch is applied, some patients require a patch change every 48 hours; should not be given to opioid naïve patients

    vii. Spinal: via indwelling catheters into the epidural or intrathecal space; an implantable pump should be used in only carefully selected patients after appropriate consultation; cost, care issues, and potential adverse effects should also be carefully weighed however can dramatically improve some patients' quality of life especially with severe pain in lower extremities

d) Adjuvant analgesics: drugs that have a primary indication other than pain (e.g., antidepressant or anticonvulsant) but are also analgesic for some painful conditions

    (1) For treatment of neuropathic pain

        i. Tricyclic antidepressants

            1. Desipramine and nortriptyline recommended over amitriptyline, which has more anticholinergic effects (causing cardiovascular changes, dry mouth, constipation)

            2. Serotonin selective reuptake inhibitors (SSRIs) have not been well studied in neuropathic pain and may seem to have limited analgesic effect

            3. Guidelines for monitoring

                a. These drugs may cause sedation and enhance sleep

                b. Response may be delayed by 3–7 days

c. Monitor adverse effects

d. Adverse effects: sedation, orthostatic hypotension, anticholinergic side effects (including urinary retention), cardiac effects

ii. Anticonvulsants

1. Most useful for lancinating, paroxysmal pain and pain that does not respond to antidepressant therapy; dose as with seizures; most experience has been with carbamazepine

2. Gabapentin (300–1800 mg TID); carbamazepine (100–800 mg BID or QID); phenytoin (100–200 mg TID); valproic acid (200–400 mg BID or TID); clonazepam (0.25–0.5 mg TID); (all doses are PO)

3. Guidelines for monitoring

   a. Watch for side effects

   b. Monitor carbamazepine, phenytoin and valproic acid serum levels for signs of toxicity

4. Major adverse effects

   a. Gabapentin: sedation, side effects generally less than with others (has less bone marrow suppression: drug of choice for patients on chemotherapy); costly

   b. Carbamazepine: bone marrow suppression, vertigo, confusion, sedation

   c. Phenytoin: ataxia, rash, hepatotoxicity

   d. Valproic acid: nausea, vomiting, sedation, ataxia, tremor, thrombocytopenia, neutropenia, hepatotoxicity

   e. Clonazepam: sedation, physical dependence

iii. Local anesthetics

1. Useful in refractory neuropathic pain

2. Lidocaine, given IV (more likely to be offered outside hospice program); tocainide (Tonocard®) and mexiletine (Mexiletine®), given orally. Mexiletine must be titrated very slowly and serum levels monitored

3. Adverse effects include dizziness, lightheadedness, lowered blood pressure, sensory disturbances and tremor, seizures at high doses, nausea and vomiting

4. Lidocaine 5% is also available in a patch for topical relief of post-herpetic neuropathy, post-thoracotomy pain and other pain syndromes

   a. The patches should be placed over intact skin only

   b. Up to three patches can be used to cover the painful area and are left in place for 12 hours, with 12 hours off

   c. Adverse effects are uncommon and include pain with removal of the patch

               d. Patients with sensitivity to touch (also called allodynia) often report relief

            iv. Baclofen (muscle relaxant): used to treat a variety of neuropathic pain problems

      (2) Corticosteroids: used in metastatic bone pain (triple effect of pain control, mood elevation and increased appetite)

      (3) Topical capsaicin: may be used for diabetic neuropathy, post-herpetic neuralgia, arthritis and Kaposi's sarcoma lesions though there are newer medications that are more effective and do not cause irritation and pain when applied

      (4) Other medications used to treat side effects of opioids (e.g., psychostimulants, phenothiazines, and benzodiazepines for muscle spasms)

B. **Non-pharmacologic interventions can be used concurrently with pharmacological and other modalities to relieve pain and can often be taught to patients and/or family members; there are some who believe that medications should never be given without the addition of <u>some</u> non-pharmacologic intervention. However, the use of non-pharmacologic interventions should <u>never</u> preclude appropriate use of medications, including opioids. The most common non-pharmacologic interventions are listed below**

   1. Physical modalities

      a) Consider physical therapy (PT) and occupational therapy (OT) consults (especially in the inpatient palliative care setting)

      b) Cutaneous stimulation (heat, cold)

      c) Exercise (with limitations based on physical condition)

      d) Transcutaneous nerve stimulation (efficacy controversial may be useful in patients with mild pain); acupuncture

      e) Massage; healing touch; therapeutic touch

   2. Psychosocial and spiritual interventions (helpful in maintaining control in uncertain, dependent and anxiety-provoking situations)

      a) Relaxation and guided imagery

      b) Distraction

      c) Music

      d) Reframing

      e) Patient and family education

      f) Hypnosis

      g) Counseling

      h) Prayer

      i) Spiritual reflection or meditation

   3. Other

      a) Biofeedback

      b) Aromatherapy

4. Palliative radiation therapy

   a) May be used to relieve symptoms of patients with advanced disease, (e.g., pain, bleeding), compression of vital organ systems (e.g., the brain, ulcerating skin lesions), and metastasis to weight bearing bones susceptible to fracture

   b) Radiation therapy is the treatment of choice for spinal cord compression, bone pain and is frequently used in superior vena cava syndrome and symptomatic brain metastases

   c) While external beam radiation is the modality commonly used for palliative radiation therapy, Strontium-89 and Samarium Sm-153 are intravenous radionucleotides that emit beta radiation at the bony metastatic site, is sometimes used to treat areas of painful skeletal metastasis; newer radionucleotides are currently under study that may not produce the painful flare that occurs when Strontium-89 is given

5. Palliative chemotherapy: may improve or enhance comfort when neither cure nor control is possible

   a) Antineoplastic therapy may produce tumor shrinkage, relief of pressure on nerves, lymphatics, and blood vessels and reduction in organ obstruction, thus relieving pain

   b) Bisphosphonates are useful in treating pain related to multiple myeloma and metastatic bone disease[2]

IV. Pain during the Final Days of Life

A. Pain Assessment

1. Patients may become nonverbal in the final days of life

   a) A furrowed brow may indicate pain

   b) Guarding and vocalization during turning or dressing changes may suggest pain

   c) A therapeutic trial of an opioid should be strongly considered to determine if these behaviors change with the use of an analgesic

2. If the patient had pain prior to becoming unresponsive, assume pain is still present

B. Pharmacologic Management

1. As organ system dysfunction increases, particularly renal clearance, drugs or their metabolites are cleared from the body less efficiently and sedation may increase

   a) Therefore, a therapeutic trial of opioid dose reduction may be indicated if sedation is not a desired effect

   b) In some cases, patients may become more alert and responsive

   c) If any signs of pain return, the dose should be returned to its previous level

2. Rapid discontinuation of opioids, benzodiazepines or other agents can result in the abstinence syndrome; whenever possible, gradual reduction in dose of these drugs is indicated

3. Sedation at the end of life is an option for patients with intractable pain and suffering[2]

   a) There are numerous combinations of medications that are used to accomplish sedation

      (1) Opioids

      (2) Barbiturates

      (3) Neuroleptics

      (4) Benzodiazepines

   b) Therapy is based on obtaining initial relief of symptoms followed by ongoing sedation to maintain the effect

   c) Parenteral ketamine, given either as a continuous infusion or as bolus doses, may also be used to accomplish sedation at the end of life

C. **Non-pharmacologic Management Should Continue**

V. **Summary of Principles of Pain Management**

A. **Pain assessment data is documented so the pain etiology or syndrome can be identified and appropriately treated**

B. **The oral route is used whenever possible**

   1. If the patient is unable to take oral medications, buccal, sublingual, rectal, and transdermal routes are considered before parenteral routes

   2. IM route is avoided

   3. IV and subcutaneous route can be used for any patient that cannot tolerate above choices under oral route or when pain is rapidly escalating and severe. Subcutaneous route is a useful alternative in the home setting when reliable IV access is not possible

C. **Constant pain calls for treatment with an around-the-clock scheduled long-acting opioid and a short-acting medication for breakthrough pain**

   1. Only one long-acting opioid is ordered for constant pain

   2. Doses of opioids are increased commensurate with the patient's report of pain

   3. Equianalgesic conversions are used when changing medications and/or routes

   4. Adjuvant medications are used for neuropathic pain, some visceral pain states, and bone pain

D. **Breakthrough pain**

   1. Only one analgesic is ordered for breakthrough pain. Ideally the same drug should be used for breakthrough pain as long acting if available (e.g., long acting MS Contin® and MSIR® for breakthrough pain)

2. A higher dosage of breakthrough, or rescue medication, is sometimes necessary if the frequency of breakthrough pain and/or intensity are at higher levels; this dose will be determined by the physician with the assistance of the registered nurse and pharmacist

3. Patients and families need to be educated about taking the medication when the pain is first perceived; not when it has become severe or unbearable

E. **Non-pharmacologic approaches are always a part of any pain management plan**

F. **An appropriate preventative bowel regimen is ordered with a stimulant laxative and stool softener to correct the effects of the opioid (see Chapter V)**

VI. **Evaluation: pain management is predicated by ongoing assessment of treatment efficacy and control of treatment side effects**

    A. **Evaluation of interventions is a basic nursing function and completes the nursing process; all nursing personnel contribute in this function**

    B. **Nursing evaluation should be accomplished in a timely manner, in accordance with expected pharmacologic peak action or when the non-pharmacologic intervention is completed**

    C. **At each nursing contact with a patient assess for**

        1. Pain intensity, type, duration, etc.

        2. Medication side effects, interactions or complications

        3. Patient's satisfaction with method of pain relief

    D. **In the inpatient setting**

        1. Pain assessment every shift or more frequently as indicated

        2. Patient and family teaching and reinforcement of pain management

        3. Monitor fluid intake, activity tolerance and bowel status daily and document

    E. **Evaluate efficacy of pain relief interventions**

        1. At appropriate intervals after any change in medication, dosage, route of administration, etc.

        2. At each nursing contact with a patient

Table 1: Pain Terms Associated with Neuropathic Pain States

(modified from the International Association for the Study of Pain; McCaffery and Pasero)

Term	Definition	
Allodynia	Pain due to a stimulus, which does not normally provoke pain	
Dysesthesia	An unpleasant abnormal sensation, whether spontaneous or evoked	
Hyperalgesia	A painful syndrome characterized by an abnormally painful reaction to a normally non-painful stimulus, such as touch (sometimes referred to as hyperpathia)	
Paresthesia	An abnormal anesthetic sensation (often described as a painful numbness)	
Neuralgia	Pain in the distribution of a nerve or nerves	
Neuropathic pain	Pain initiated or caused by a primary lesion or dysfunction in the nervous system	
	Peripheral neuropathic pain	Pain initiated or caused by a primary lesion or dysfunction in the peripheral nervous system (e.g., postherpetic neuropathy)
	Central pain	Pain initiated or caused by a primary lesion or dysfunction in the central nervous system (e.g., post-thalamic pain syndrome occurring after stroke)

Table 2: Combination Products

Opioid	Proprietary name and combination drugs[a]
Hydrocodone	Vicodin® (5 mg + 500 mg acetaminophen) Vicodin ES® (7.5 mg + 750 mg acetaminophen) Lorcet-10® (10 mg + 650 mg acetaminophen) Lortab® (5 or 10 mg + 500 mg acetaminophen) Vicodin HP® (10 mg + 660 mg acetaminophen) Norco® (5, 7.5 or 10 mg + 325 mg acetaminophen) Anexsia® (5 mg + 500 mg acetaminophen) Zydone® (5 mg + 400 mg acetaminophen) Vicoprofen® (7.5 mg + 200 mg ibuprofen) Reprexain™ (5 mg + 200 mg ibuprofen)
Oxycodone	Percodan® (5 mg + 325 mg ASA) Percocet® (5 mg + 325 mg acetaminophen) Tylox® (5 mg + 500 mg acetaminophen) Roxicet® (5 mg + 325 mg acetaminophen) Combunox™ (5 mg + 400 mg ibuprofen)
Codeine	Tylenol #2® (15 mg + 325 mg acetaminophen) Tylenol #3® (30 mg + 325 mg acetaminophen) Tylenol #4® (60 mg + 325 mg acetaminophen)
Propoxyphene[b]	Darvon® (65 mg) Darvocet N® (100 mg + 650 mg acetaminophen) Darvon Compound® (65 mg + 325 mg ASA + caffeine) Darvon-N® or Darvon® with ASA (65 mg + 325 mg ASA)

[a] Twenty-four hour dose of acetaminophen should not exceed 4 grams for healthy adults, less than 3 grams for persons with liver dysfunction, or who are elderly.

[b] WARNING: Long-lived metabolite that is toxic to the central nervous system and cardiovascular system, not recommended for long-term use and use in the elderly.

Cited References

1. McCaffery M, Pasero C. *Pain: Clinical Manual*. St. Louis, MO: Mosby; 1999.
2. Paice JA, Fine P. Pain at the end of life. In: Ferrell B, Coyle N, eds. *Textbook of Palliative Nursing*. New York, NY: Oxford University Press; 2006:131–153.
3. Coyle N, Layman-Goldstein M. Pain assessment and pharmacological/nonpharmacological interventions. In: Matzo M, Sherman DW, eds. *Palliative Care Nursing: Quality Care to the End of Life*. New York, NY: Springer Publishing Company; 2010:357–410.
4. World Health Organization. *Cancer: Palliative Care*. Available at: http://www.who.int/cancer/palliative/en/. Accessed February 3, 2010.
5. Lussier D, Portenoy R. Adjuvant analgesics in pain management. In: Doyle D, Hanks G, Cherny NI, Calman K, eds. *Oxford Textbook of Palliative Medicine*. 3rd ed. New York, NY: Oxford University Press; 2005:349–378.
6. Benjamin LJ, Dampler CD, Jacox A, et al. *Guidelines for the Management of Acute and Chronic Pain in Sickle-Cell Disease*. Skokie, IL: American Pain Society; 1999.
7. Cleeland CS, Gonin R, Hatfield AK, et al. Pain and its treatment in outpatients with metastatic cancer. *New England Journal of Medicine*. 1994;330:592–596.
8. Fairchild A. Undertreatment of cancer pain. *Curr Opin Support Palliat Care*. 2010;4(1):11–15.
9. Anderson KO, Green CR, Payne R. Racial and ethnic disparities in pain: causes and consequences of unequal care. *J Pain*. 2009;10(12):1187–1204.

Additional References and Resources

AGS Panel on the Pharmacological Management of Persistent Pain in Older Persons. *AGS Clinical Practice Guideline: Pharmacological Management of Persistent Pain in Older Persons*. 2009. Available at: www.americangeriatrics.org/education/pharm_management.shtml.

American Medical Directors Association (AMDA). *Clinical Practice Guideline: Pain Management*. Columbia, MD: American Medical Directors Association; 2009.

American Pain Society. *Principles of Analgesic Use in the Treatment of Acute Pain and Cancer Pain*. 6th ed. Skokie, IL: American Pain Society; 2008.

Heiskanen T, Haakana S, Gergov M, et al. Transdermal fentanyl in cachectic cancer patients. *Pain*. 2009;144(1–2):218–222.

McPherson ML, Kaiser KS, Burns C. Interpretation and implementation of range, titration, and prn orders in hospice. *Journal of Hospice and Palliative Nursing*. 2005;7(5):289–298.

Mehta A, Chan LS. Understanding of the concept of "total pain": a prerequisite for pain control. *Journal of Hospice and Palliative Nursing*. 2008;10(1):26–32.

Panke JT. Difficulties in managing pain at the end of life. *Journal of Hospice and Palliative Nursing*. 2002;5(2):83–90.

Rosenfield RL, Stahl D. Pain management of bone metastases in breast cancer. *Journal of Hospice and Palliative Nursing.* 2006;8(4):233–244.

Shaver WA. Suffering and the role of abandonment of self. *Journal of Hospice and Palliative Nursing.* 2002;4(1):46–53.

SUPPORT Study Principal Investigators. A controlled trial to improve care for seriously ill hospitalized patients: a study to understand prognoses and preferences for outcomes and risks of treatments (SUPPORT). *Journal of the American Medical Association.* 1995;274:1591–1598.

Weissman DE, Griffie J, Muchka S, Matson S. Building an institutional commitment to pain management in long term care facilities. *Journal of Pain and Symptom Management.* 2000;20:35–43.

Wrede-Seaman L. *Symptom Management Algorithms: A Handbook for Palliative Care.* 3rd ed. Yakima, WA: Intellicard; 2009.

Zerwekh J, Riddell S, Richard J. Fearing to comfort: a grounded theory of constraints to opioid use in hospice. *Journal of Hospice and Palliative Nursing.* 2002;4(2):83–90.

Chapter V

Symptom Management

Roger Strong, PhD, RN, ACHNP®, FPCN

Adapted from: Collins CA, Wilson MA. Symptom management. In: Volker BG, Watson AC, eds. *Core Curriculum for the Generalist Hospice and Palliative Nurse*. Dubuque, IA: Kendall Hunt Publishing; 2002:89–154.

I. Principles

    A. The nursing process (using assessment, diagnosis, planning, for symptom management and care at the end of life)

    B. Care at the end of life is multidimensional with emphasis on quality of life as the patient and family define it, with respect for, support and education of patient and family

    C. Understanding of expectations, goals of treatment, end-of-life goals. Issues must be clarified with patient and family, taking into account the patient's position on the disease trajectory. Remember that goals change over time and patients and families may change their mind as to which interventions they want over time as the disease progresses

    D. The interdisciplinary team (IDT) is the framework for palliative care and hospice

    E. The patient and family are the unit of care in palliative care and hospice and are included in the assessment, planning, decision-making, and evaluation of interventions

        1. Options and expected or possible outcomes are discussed with patient and family to inform their decision-making; the IDT is responsible for giving them information regarding the benefits and the burdens of any treatment that is proposed

        2. Patients and families require time, opportunity for clarification, and review in anticipation of making decisions

    F. The end of life can be a time of growth, reconciliation, peace, joy and hope for patients and families; appropriate symptom management can facilitate this process by maximizing patient comfort

G. **Authors' note: patients may experience a variety of symptoms. Those covered in this chapter are some of the most often experienced by individuals with life-threatening illness**

II. **Alteration in Skin and Mucous Membranes**

   A. **Definition: disruption in the integrity of the skin or oral mucous membrane**

   B. **Possible Etiologies**
   1. Skin integrity
      a) Pressure ulcers
         (1) Pressure to the skin, causing a decrease in blood flow and eventual cell death
         (2) Shearing forces, in which two surfaces slide in opposite but parallel directions (e.g., a patient slides down in bed and bone and skin are displaced from one another)
         (3) Friction, in which two surfaces move across one another (e.g., patient is dragged across bed sheets)
         (4) Moisture (especially feces and urine)
         (5) Obesity
         (6) Malnutrition
         (7) Immobility
         (8) Impaired circulation due to peripheral vascular disease, diabetes or cancer infiltration through skin
      b) Fistulas
      c) Tumor necrosis
   2. Alteration of oral mucous membranes
      a) Dry mouth (xerostomia)
         (1) Candidiasis
         (2) Drugs (anticholinergics, antihistamines, phenothiazines)
         (3) Radiation and chemotherapy
         (4) Dehydration
         (5) Mucositis
         (6) Mouth breathing
         (7) Metabolic disorders (hypercalcemia, hyperglycemia)
      b) Candidiasis
         (1) Radiation and chemotherapy
         (2) Drugs (antibiotics, corticosteroids)

- c) Herpes simplex virus
- d) Mucositis caused by radiation or chemotherapy

3. Pruritus: uncomfortable itching of the skin
   - a) Dry, flaky skin
   - b) Wet, macerated skin
   - c) Contact dermatitis caused by ointments or creams
   - d) Infestations caused by scabies, lice, fleas
   - e) Drugs (antibiotics, morphine, phenothiazines)
   - f) Systemic disease (renal failure, hepatobiliary disease, infiltration of tumors into subcutaneous tissue)
   - g) Fungal infections

C. **Assess for**
   1. Skin integrity
      - a) Inspect skin each time patient changes position
      - b) If pressure ulcer, grade wound according to stage[1]
         - (1) Stage I: non-blanchable erythema of intact skin, the heralding lesion of skin ulceration
            - i. In individuals with dark skin, discoloration of the skin, warmth, edema, induration or hardness also may be indicators
            - ii. Skin changes may be difficult to discern in some persons of color and the patient's report of pain may be the only cue to closely examine at-risk areas; be mindful of baseline skin color and monitor skin frequently for skin color change
         - (2) Stage II: partial thickness skin loss involving epidermis, dermis, or both. The ulcer is superficial and presents clinically as an abrasion, blister or shallow crater
         - (3) Stage III: full thickness skin loss involving damage to or necrosis of subcutaneous tissue that may extend down to, but not through, underlying fascia. The ulcer presents clinically as a deep crater with or without undermining of adjacent tissue
         - (4) Stage IV: full thickness skin loss with extensive destruction, tissue necrosis, or damage to muscle, bone, or supporting structures; undermining and sinus tracts also may be associated with Stage IV pressure ulcers
      - c) Wound location
      - d) Wound appearance
         - (1) Size, length, width, depth, undermining
         - (2) Presence of drainage (serous, serosanguineous, sanguineous, purulent) and amount

(3) Tissue type (i.e., granulating or eschar)

(4) Appearance of surrounding skin (redness, maceration, etc.)

e) Is wound painful?

f) If wound is due to tumor necrosis, does the location present a potential for serious complications (i.e., potential for hemorrhage or obstruction of blood flow due to the tumor located next to blood vessels)?

g) Is the wound malodorous or fungating?

h) A nutritional assessment is important, as malnutrition can impede proper wound healing and also cause pressure ulcer formation

2. Alteration in oral mucous membranes

a) Patient history of mouth dryness or sore mouth

b) Review of medications which may cause oral membrane alterations (i.e., antibiotics, chemotherapy drugs such as IV 5-Fluouracil, anticholinergics)

c) Examination of internal and external oral mucosa

(1) Dry, cracked lips

(2) Sores or white patches on buccal membranes, oropharynx or tongue

(3) Bleeding of gums, lips or tongue

d) Patient's current oral hygiene regimen

e) Patient and family knowledge of etiology and management of altered oral mucous membranes

3. Pruritus

a) History of itching (including when, how long, what is tolerable)

b) Assessment of skin

(1) Presence of rashes or lesions

(2) Presence of abrasions from frequent scratching

(3) Overall skin integrity

c) Review plan of care for medications that may cause pruritus

D. Diagnoses

1. Impaired skin integrity, oral, related to dry mouth, oral lesions, infection

2. Impaired skin integrity related to immobility and pressure over bony prominences

3. Impaired skin integrity related to tumor necrosis or fistula

4. Pain related to altered skin or oral mucous membranes or pruritus

5. Body image disturbance related to malodorous or unsightly wounds

6. Patient and family knowledge deficit related to etiology and management of wounds, altered oral mucous membranes, or pruritus

E. **Planning and Intervention**

1. Wound management

    a) Relieve pressure

        (1) Turn at least every two hours

        (2) Place patient on pressure relief and pressure reduction support surfaces

    b) Reduce friction and shearing forces

        (1) Teach family proper techniques for moving patient in bed; physical therapy referral may be indicated

        (2) Use transparent dressings or elbow and knee protectors

    c) Consult team dietitian for nutritional assessment and plan of care

    d) Consult enterostomal therapy (ET) nurse for wound management plan, if appropriate

    e) Consult Agency for Healthcare Research and Quality (AHRQ) (formerly AHCPR) guidelines for skin and wound care

    f) Wounds should be cleansed and irrigated with normal saline prior to being dressed

        (1) Dressing selection

            i. The following should be considered when selecting a dressing[1]

                1. Moist wound bed

                2. Dry surrounding skin

                3. Exudate control

                4. Caregiver time

            ii. If wounds are malodorous, special dressings are required to assist with odor control

                1. Metronidazole tablets crushed and sprinkled into the malodorous wound will help minimize infection and odor

            iii. Table 1 lists different types of dressings and the types of wounds for which they are appropriate

        (2) Assure adequate pain control prior to changing dressings; utilize topical pain relievers as appropriate for ongoing pain (i.e., topical lidocaine, cold packs)

2. Alteration in oral mucous membranes

    a) Xerostomia

        (1) Stimulate salivation

            i. Peppermint water

            ii. Gum, mints, hard candy (preferably sugar free to protect teeth)

            iii. Ice chips or frequent sips of water

iv. Pilocarpine 2.5 mg PO TID, titrate to 10 mg PO TID; do not use in patients with severe COPD or bowel obstruction[2]

    b) Utilize saliva substitutes

        (1) Ice chips or frequent sips of water

        (2) Artificial saliva

    c) Treat dehydration

        (1) Ice chips or frequent sips of water

        (2) Offer fluids throughout the day, especially with meals

        (3) Humidify the room

        (4) Place spray bottle and moistened oral swabs close to patient (avoid lemon-glycerin swabs)

    d) Review medications, and alter regimen if appropriate

3. Sore mouth due to oral Candida, herpetic lesions, mucositis or stomatitis

    a) For Candida, nystatin swish and swallow or fluconazole tablets or suspension

    b) Around-the-clock mouth care at least every two to four hours with moistened oral swabs and saline mouth rinse, if patient is able; be sure to apply water-soluble lubricant to lips

    c) 1:4 hydrogen peroxide and water rinse for mucous or hard debris in mouth[3]

    d) Do not serve hot or overly spicy foods; serve softened and moist foods rather than dry

    e) Several oral medications and medicated mouthwash cocktails are available for mouth pain and lesions. Some examples are

        (1) Topical morphine

        (2) Viscous lidocaine

        (3) Cocktail of Milk of Magnesia, diphenhydrAMINE, and viscous lidocaine

        (4) Sucralfate slurry

4. Pruritus interventions

    a) Non-pharmacologic measures

        (1) Avoid skin irritants that may cause dryness or additional moisture[4]

            i. Alcohol

            ii. Tight or heavy clothing

            iii. Frequent bathing with harsh soaps and hot water

        (2) Avoid heat, maintain cool room temperatures; keep the patient cool to avoid sweating, and frequently cleanse the skin with neutral pH cleansers and tepid water

        (3) Cool starch baths

(4) Cold compresses can decrease itching; make sure to assess skin frequently during application, and do not apply if patient's peripheral vascular system is compromised

(5) Apply lubricating ointments or creams to skin (i.e., lanolin, Udder Cream®) to avoid excessive drying

(6) Avoid alcohol, foods/drinks containing caffeine, theophylline

b) Pharmacologic measures

(1) Antihistamines such as hydroxyzine and diphenhydrAMINE

(2) Topical corticosteroids can be used for acute localized itching, but should be avoided for chronic pruritus[4]

(3) Ondansetron and cholestyramine have been used in cholestatic, uremic, and opioid-induced pruritus[4]

(4) Antifungal creams for pruritus related to Candida

(5) Transcutaneous electrical nerve stimulation (TENS) units may be helpful in localized pruritus[3,4]

F. Patient and Family Education

1. Wounds

   a) Demonstrate correct positioning to maximize pressure relief. Explain importance of changing patient's position every two hours, when appropriate, even if the patient is sitting in a chair

   b) Demonstrate proper technique in moving patient up in bed to reduce friction and shearing force

   c) Demonstrate correct procedures for cleansing and dressing wounds

   d) Explain possible complications with tumor necrotic wounds; prepare family for bleeding or airway concerns and management

   e) Explain management of ostomy bags if fistula present

2. Altered oral mucous membranes

   a) Demonstrate proper technique for oral care; explain importance of frequent oral care

   b) Explain medication usage and potential side effects

   c) Introduce non-pharmacologic methods for preventing and relieving dry and sore oral mucous membranes

3. Pruritus

   a) Explain etiology of pruritus

   b) Explain ways of preventing pruritus (keep skin clean and dry, avoid soaps, etc.)

   c) Explain actions of medications and potential side effects

   d) Introduce non-pharmacologic methods for preventing and relieving pruritus (See Section E, 4 a) above)

G. Evaluate
1. Wounds
   a) Response of patient and family to teaching
   b) Effectiveness of interventions (i.e., is wound healing?)
   c) Need for change in plan (i.e., change in dressing, referral to ET nurse)
   d) Patient and family understanding of treatment and prevention of further alteration of skin integrity
2. Altered oral mucous membranes and pruritus
   a) Response to interventions and patient and family teaching
   b) Effectiveness of interventions: are patient and family satisfied with outcome?
   c) Medication effects and side effects
   d) Patient and family understanding of treatment and prevention of further alteration

H. Revise plan according to findings from ongoing evaluations, changes in patient status, or family needs

Table 1: Indications and Uses for Dressings

Type of Dressing	Indications and Uses
Semipermeable film	Protects very early damage from shear forces Prevents bacterial contamination Maintains humidity in shallow ulcers, producing ideal conditions for granulation and healing Provides immediate pain relief Best applied when there is no exudation from the wound
Hydrocolloids	For low-exudate wounds Maintains moist environment Fluidizes to produce a gel useful for debridement Provides environment for granulation Available as a paste to fill wound cavities
Alginates	For heavy exudates; controls secretion and bacterial contamination by absorption and formation of hydrophilic gel
Hydrogels/xerogels	For debridement in the presence of slough and infection: rehydrates eschar and makes it easier to remove
Enzymatic	For eschar and necrotic tissue; loosens necrotic tissue by liquefaction, thereby aiding in its removal (Protect edges of wound with zinc paste and apply to eschar under an occlusive dressing)
Polysaccharide dextranomer	For exudative, infected wounds; on contact with wound exudates the beads absorb fluid and swell, forming a gel; bacteria and dead cells are drawn away from the wound. Applied every 24 hours until wound is clean and granulation tissue is developing
Charcoal	Malodorous infected pressure sores: adsorbs bacteria, cellular debris, toxins, and odors

Reprinted with permission from: Waller A, Caroline NL. *Handbook of Palliative Care in Cancer.* 2nd ed. Boston, MA: Butterworth-Heinemann; 2000:97.

III. **Altered Mental Status: Confusion, Delirium, Terminal Restlessness, Agitation**

    A.   Confusion/Delirium/Agitation

        1.   Definitions

            a)   Confusion

                (1)   Clouding of consciousness, memory impairment

                (2)   Change in cognition/impaired cognitive function, impaired perceptions and emotional disturbances

                (3)   May be accompanied by reduced level of consciousness, disorientation, and misperceptions

b) Delirium

    (1) Exaggerated emotions or memories with aggression, paranoia, or terror displayed

    (2) Disturbance of consciousness with reduced ability to focus

    (3) Disturbance develops over a short period of time (hours or days) and tends to fluctuate over the course of the day

c) Agitation

    (1) Can occur at any time during a disease process and is an objective result of confusion or delirium

    (2) A group of symptoms that may include physically and/or verbally aggressive behaviors, hiding or hoarding behaviors and physically non-aggressive behaviors (i.e., pacing, inappropriate dressing/undressing, repetitive actions)[5]

2. Potential etiologies

    a) Medications: opioids, phenothiazines, benzodiazepines, anticholinergics, beta-blockers, diuretics, dopaminergics, steroids, atropine, phenytoin, H_2 antagonists, digoxin only when toxic

    b) Unrelieved pain, discomfort or other unrelieved symptoms

    c) Full bladder or bowel

    d) Infection (UTI, lung, septicemia)

    e) Brain tumor, primary or metastatic

    f) Cardiac or respiratory failure

    g) Metabolic disturbance (calcium, urea nitrogen, glucose, sodium)

    h) Nicotine, alcohol, drug withdrawal

    i) Extreme, uncontrolled anxiety

    j) Posttraumatic stress disorder (PTSD)

3. Assess for

    a) Confusion vs. delirium using available tools such as those listed below[5]

        (1) Memorial Delirium Assessment Scale (MDAS)

        (2) Delirium Rating Scale (DRS)

        (3) NEECHAM Confusion Scale (NCS)

        (4) Confusion Assessment Method (CAM)

    b) Differentiation between hyper-alert—hyperactive and hypo-alert—hypoactive variants of delirium

    c) Patient's previous personality and emotional coping abilities

    d) Alcohol, drug use history; recent nicotine, alcohol or drug use

e) Signs of infection

　　(1) Fever, flushing, tachycardia, tachypnea, perspiration

　　(2) These symptoms of infection may not be present in persons with immunosuppression due to corticosteroids, chemotherapy, disease process or in the elderly

f) Abdominal examination: palpate for bladder or bowel, abdominal distention

g) Bowel history, noting time and character of last bowel movement; rectal examination for impaction

h) If diabetic history or currently on corticosteroids, capillary blood glucose

i) Lab studies including: BUN, creatinine, electrolytes, glucose, calcium

j) Consider midstream clean-catch urinalysis, culture, and sensitivity

k) Neurologic status: dysphasia, weakness, bilateral strength, coordination; poor coordination

l) Patient safety

m) Patient and family coping with change in mental status and ways of managing patient

4. Potential diagnoses

　　a) Altered mental status changes potentially related to (etiology)

　　b) High safety risk for fall related to altered mental status

　　c) Impaired bowel function related to constipation from (etiology)

　　d) Impaired bladder function related to retention from (etiology)

　　e) Disturbed physiologic response to infection related to corticosteroid use, aging

　　f) Impaired physiologic response related to alcohol, drugs, medication

　　g) Risk for alcohol, drug withdrawal due to recent use

5. Planning and intervention

　　a) Etiology of altered mental status will determine intervention plan

　　b) Effective pain control and control of other disabling symptoms

　　c) Assess patient's current medications for compliance, effects and iatrogenic effects (side effects) contributing to altered mental status

　　d) Review with physician and/or pharmacist; consider discontinuation or reduction of medications thought to be contributing to patient's confusion

　　e) Correct metabolic imbalance, if appropriate

　　f) Support alcohol, drug withdrawal chemically as indicated

　　g) Treat infection as appropriate

　　h) For impaction, disimpact; establish aggressive bowel regimen

　　i) For urine retention, straight or retention catheter to relieve

- j) Support withdrawal from nicotine, alcohol or drugs if withdrawal is contributing to agitation
- k) Reassure patient and family and provide constant, consistent reorientation of confused patient
- l) Provide for patient's safety; follow agency/institutional policy regarding the use of restraints, both chemical and physical
- m) Avoid sedation if possible
- n) Psychotropic drugs do not reverse confusion or altered mental status, but they may calm distressing agitation, paranoia or hallucinations
  - (1) Haloperidol and chlorpromazine are first line medications
  - (2) Risperidone is particularly helpful in managing agitation and hallucinations in the elderly

6. Patient and family education
   - a) Since confusion is most distressing to patients and families, much education and support is required
   - b) Intermittent nature of most confusion
   - c) Expected therapeutic response to interventions
   - d) Expected medication effects and potential side effects
   - e) Safety needs of patient during periods of confusion, agitation
   - f) Importance of compliance with bowel regimen, bladder emptying

7. Evaluate
   - a) Effectiveness of interventions
     - (1) Medications
     - (2) Non-pharmacologic interventions
   - b) Family participation and coping
   - c) Reassess to determine additional needs

8. Revise plan according to findings from ongoing evaluations, changes in patient status, or family needs

B. Terminal Restlessness

1. Definitions
   - a) Excessive restlessness, increased mental and physical activity[5]
   - b) Commonly seen features are frequent, non-purposeful motor activity, inability to concentrate or relax, disturbances in sleep or rest patterns, potential for progression to agitation[7]

2. Potential etiologies include

    a) Full bladder, constipation/impaction

    b) Hypoxia, dyspnea

    c) Left ventricular failure, decreased cardiac output

    d) Uncontrolled pain

    e) Denial, anxiety, unfinished emotional, and/or spiritual issues

    f) Also consider the possible etiologies listed above for confusion/delirium/agitation

3. Assess for

    a) Etiology of terminal restlessness

    b) Emotional, spiritual history related to issues, personal peace, resolution

    c) Shortness of breath or labored breathing; lung sounds

    d) Bladder and bowel status

    e) Hallucinations, muscle twitching or jerking

    f) "Sundowning"

4. Potential diagnoses

    a) Disturbed mental status related to (etiology)

    b) High risk for injury due to agitation and uncontrolled restlessness

    c) Family coping impairment related to severe stress of uncontrolled agitation

5. Plan and interventions

    a) Etiology of restlessness will determine intervention plan

    b) Disimpaction, bladder relief if distended

    c) Consult physician or pharmacist for pharmacologic management. Medications may include

        (1) Opioid analgesics for pain and sedation

        (2) Antipsychotics

            i. ChlorproMAZINE

            ii. Haloperidol

            iii. Risperidone is particularly helpful in managing agitation and hallucinations in the elderly

        (3) Barbiturates

            i. Phenobarbital

(4) Benzodiazepines

　　i. Lorazepam (if no delirium, caution with dementia)

　　ii. Diazepam (caution with dementia)

　　iii. Midazolam

d) Medications should be given by the least invasive route possible: oral, rectal, transdermal, subcutaneous or intravenous; intramuscular route should be used only if absolutely necessary

e) Regular assessment of medication effects

f) Pharmacologic control of muscle twitching, jerking

g) Pastoral and psychological support of patient and family for emotional and spiritual issues

h) Non-pharmacologic approaches including

(1) Subdued, quiet, calm environment

(2) Consistent, familiar faces, and staff

(3) Calm and reassuring presence

(4) Relaxation techniques

　　i. Visualization

　　ii. Distraction

　　iii. Massage

(5) Pet therapy, if appropriate

(6) Aromatherapy

6. Family education

a) Calm environment, presence with minimal stimulation

b) Non-pharmacologic methods for cueing patient with relaxation, visualization, massage, music, distraction

c) Expected therapeutic response to medications and potential side effects

d) Prepare family for patient's sedation response to medications

e) Prepare family for patient's death; encourage speaking with/to patient and using "letting go" language and phrases if family able

7. Evaluate

a) Effectiveness of interventions

(1) Medications

(2) Non-pharmacologic interventions

b) Family participation and coping

c) Reassess to determine additional needs

8. Revise plan according to findings from ongoing evaluations, changes in patient status, or family needs

IV. **Anorexia and Cachexia**

   A. **Definitions**
      1. Anorexia: loss of appetite or inability to take in nutrients
      2. Cachexia: weight loss and wasting due to inadequate intake of nutrients

   B. **Possible Etiologies**
      1. Anorexia
         a) Pain
         b) Constipation
         c) Nausea and vomiting
         d) Alteration in oral mucous membranes (candidiasis, xerostomia, mucositis)
         e) Impaired gastric emptying
         f) Change of taste in foods (dysgeusia); change in smell of foods
         g) Altered mental status (depression, dementia, confusion, anxiety)
         h) Fatigue
         i) Medications (opioids, antibiotics)
         j) Radiation or chemotherapy
      2. Cachexia
         a) Increased nutritional losses related to etiologies associated with anorexia
         b) Increased nutritional losses associated with[3]
            (1) Bleeding
            (2) Diarrhea
            (3) Malabsorption of nutrients (i.e., pancreatic cancer)
         c) Metabolic disorders
            (1) Abnormal protein metabolism (negative nitrogen balance and decreased muscle mass)
            (2) Abnormal carbohydrate metabolism due to inefficient energy metabolism
            (3) Abnormal lipid metabolism (overall depletion of total body fat)
            (4) Change in fluid and electrolyte balance (increase in extracellular fluid and total body sodium and decrease in intracellular fluid and total body potassium)[3]

C. **Assess for**
  1. History of loss of appetite, including reasons for loss (i.e., change in taste or smell, dysphagia, nausea and vomiting)
  2. Patient food likes and dislikes
  3. Oral mucosa for dryness, sores, candidiasis
  4. Medications that may cause a decrease in appetite
  5. Symptoms of malabsorption, such as diarrhea
  6. Decrease in bowel sounds
  7. Signs and symptoms of constipation or fecal impaction
  8. Signs and symptoms of metabolic disorder, such as hypoglycemia, hypernatremia, hypokalemia, dehydration, hypercalcemia
  9. Patient and family knowledge of etiology of anorexia and cachexia

D. **Potential Diagnoses**
  1. Nutrition less than body requirements related to anorexia
  2. Fatigue, related to decreased nutritional intake secondary to anorexia
  3. Body image disturbance, related to cachexia
  4. Anxiety related to inability to eat as desired
  5. Patient and family knowledge deficit related to etiology and management of anorexia/cachexia

E. **Planning and Interventions**[3]
  1. Encourage patient and family to prepare foods the patient likes and have those foods available whenever the patient requests them
  2. Refer to interdisciplinary team dietitian
  3. Give patient permission to eat less than before
  4. Encourage small, frequent meals rather than three large meals
  5. Avoid strong odors; allow food to cool before serving
  6. Serve small portions with a pleasing appearance
  7. In cases where anorexia is due to nausea/vomiting, altered oral mucous membranes, constipation, or diarrhea (see sections II, X, XI in this chapter)
  8. Encourage nutritional supplements
  9. Enteral feedings may be appropriate in certain cases if patient's gastrointestinal function is adequate for digestion/absorption
  10. Parenteral nutrition support (total or peripheral parenteral nutrition (i.e., TPN or PPN) if indicated and desired by patient and family (rare in hospice setting)
  11. Pharmacologic interventions (see Table 2)

F. **Patient and Family Education**

1. Encourage patient to eat as often as desired, but assure patient it is okay not to eat if it is uncomfortable
2. Explain dying process to patient and family, especially that anorexia is normal in last days of life
3. Encourage open communication regarding nutrition

G. **Evaluate**

1. Has patient's appetite and nutritional intake increased, if this was a goal?
2. Patient and family response to interventions. Are they satisfied with outcome?
3. Are symptoms contributing to anorexia/cachexia treated, if appropriate?

H. **Revise plan according to findings from ongoing evaluations, changes in patient status, or family needs**

Table 2: Anorexia/Cachexia: Pharmacologic Interventions

Class of Drug	Example(s)	Comments
Gastrokinetic Agents	Metoclopramide 10 mg PO TID	Useful in patients complaining of nausea or early satiety.
Corticosteroids	Dexamethasone 4 mg PO q am, then taper gradually to the minimum effective dosage	Highly effective in improving appetite in the short term, with side effects at the dosage recommended; may lose efficacy after a few weeks.
Progesterone Analogs	Megestrol acetate 400–800 mg PO QD MedroxyPROGESTERone acetate 100 mg PO TID	80% of patients will show improvement in appetite; significant decreases in nausea and vomiting occur in more than 50%; abnormalities of taste are often reduced and weight gain (of fat, fluid, and lean body mass) is seen in nearly all patients except those in the most terminal stages. Treatment with recommended dosage costs $2/day (more expensive but has fewer side effects than steroids).
Cannabinoids	Dronabinol 2.5 mg PO BID 1 hour PC	An effective appetite stimulant in low doses, without the usual side effects of drowsiness and muddled thinking.
Alcohol	1 glass of beer or sherry before meals	May improve appetite and morale in patients who enjoyed a drink before dinner when they were well.
Vitamins	Multivitamins Vitamin C, 500 mg QID	Anecdotal evidence of improved appetite (may be due to placebo effect).

Reprinted with permission from Waller A, Caroline NL. *Handbook of Palliative Care in Cancer.* 2nd ed. Boston, MA: Butterworth-Heinemann; 2000:152.

V. Ascites

    A. **Definition: the accumulation of excessive fluid in the peritoneal cavity**

    B. **Possible Etiologies**

        1. Portal hypertension: obstruction of portal vessels, causing leakage into abdominal cavity. Usually due to

            a) Cirrhosis

            b) Cancer (ovarian, endometrial, breast, colon, pancreatic, gastric, lymphoma, liver)

            c) Cardiac dysfunction: congestive heart failure, constrictive pericarditis

        2. Decreased plasma oncotic pressure: decrease in plasma albumin levels, causing fluid to leave plasma and accumulate in abdomen. Usually due to

            a) Cirrhosis

            b) Nephrotic syndrome

            c) Malnutrition

        3. Lymphatic obstruction due to tumor infiltration in the abdomen, causing a buildup of fluid in the abdomen

    C. **Assess for**

        1. History relating to etiology (i.e., liver damage, cancer, alcoholism)

        2. Weight gain

        3. Tachycardia, dyspnea, orthopnea

        4. Decrease in mobility: unable to bend or sit straight

        5. Peripheral edema

        6. Abdominal signs

            a) Measure abdominal girth every visit

            b) Fluid wave test

            c) Shifting dullness test

            d) Abdominal striae

            e) Distended abdominal wall veins

        7. Dehydration

        8. Anorexia/early satiety

    D. **Diagnoses**

        1. Pain, related to increasing abdominal girth

        2. Immobility, and fatigue secondary to ascites

3. Impaired gas exchange related to ascites

4. Activity intolerance related to ascites

5. Patient and family knowledge deficit related to etiology and treatment of ascites

E. **Planning and Intervention**

1. Treatment is determined by the extent of fluid accumulation

2. Analgesics (usually low-dose opioids) can be used for the pain and discomfort of abdominal distention

3. Fluid and sodium restriction: limit fluid to 500–1000 cc/day, and sodium to 200–1000 mg/day; may not be successful in malignant ascites[6]

4. Diuretics may be added if fluid and sodium restriction has not been successful after four to five days; spironolactone (Aldactone®) is drug of choice, with furosemide (Lasix®) added with start of spironolactone or if spironolactone alone is not successful

5. Paracentesis may be indicated for palliation if the patient's comfort is extremely compromised

6. Palliative chemotherapy may reduce tumor size and invasion, which may be causing ascites

7. Close monitoring of intake and output may be needed, depending on where patient is on disease trajectory

F. **Patient and Family Education**

1. Discuss dietary measures (fluid and sodium restriction) to reduce ascites

2. Explain effects of medication and potential side effects (including dehydration for diuretics)

3. Explain skin problems associated with ascites, and demonstrate proper measures for maintaining skin integrity

4. Discuss signs and symptoms of infection if paracentesis is part of the treatment plan

G. **Evaluate**

1. Effectiveness of interventions and patient and family teaching (are patient and family satisfied with outcome?)

2. Medication effectiveness and presence of side effects

3. Skin integrity

H. **Revise plan according to findings from ongoing evaluations, changes in patient status, or family needs**

VI. Aphasia

A. **Definition: absence or impairment of ability to communicate through speech, writing or signs**

B. **Possible Etiologies**
1. Left cerebral hemisphere lesion from infarct, hemorrhage, tumor, trauma, or degeneration
2. Advanced dementia, cerebral vascular disease

C. **Assess for**
1. Type of aphasia
    a) Sensory (receptive) aphasia: inability to comprehend spoken or written words
    b) Motor (expressive) aphasia: comprehension but inability or impairment of speech
    c) Global (sensory and motor) aphasia: failure of all forms of communication
2. Impairment of patient's ability to communicate pain, comfort needs
3. Difficulty in assessment of patient orientation, knowledge, judgment, abstraction, calculation ability and emotional responses, which can impact patient education, safety management
4. Caregiver's abilities, willingness to interpret patient's needs
5. Patient and family frustration, anxiety about deficits in communication

D. **Potential Diagnoses**
1. Speech and communication impairment related to type of aphasia and probable etiology
2. Compromised patient and family coping, stress, tolerance related to onset of aphasia
3. Patient knowledge deficit related to adjustment to impairment, disease process, therapeutic regimen related to aphasia

E. **Planning and Intervention**
1. Model acceptance and patience in communication
2. Speech therapy clinician consultation for recommendations for improving communication
3. Writing or picture boards for expressive aphasia
4. Ongoing inquiry and monitoring of patient's non-verbal behaviors for anxiety, pain, discomfort
5. Consistency in communication with patient from family and interdisciplinary team members

F. **Patient and Family Education**
1. Instruct, support caregiver/family in learning patient's non-verbal cues and developing signs, signals for communicating patient's needs (e.g., pain relief, toileting, thirst, hunger, repositioning, emotional feelings)
2. Instruct in reducing excessive stimuli in environment that can distract communication

G. **Evaluate for effectiveness of interventions, specifically**
    1. Development of alternate communication tools
    2. Patient and family coping and adaptation
    3. Patient comfort: symptom progression or relief (pain or other)
    4. Patient needs being met
    5. Interdisciplinary team consistency

H. **Revise plan according to findings from ongoing evaluations, changes in patient status, or family needs**

VII. **Bladder Spasms**

   A. **Definition: intermittent, painful contractions of the detrusor muscle, leading to suprapubic pain and urgency**

   B. **Possible Etiologies**
      1. Indwelling catheter and/or problems associated with indwelling catheters (obstruction, size or balloon too large)
      2. Urinary tract infection
      3. Encroachment on bladder or urethra by tumor or impacted feces
      4. Radiation or chemotherapy cystitis
      5. Urethral obstruction by tumors or blood clots
      6. Neurologic disorders: stroke, spinal cord lesions, multiple sclerosis

   C. **Assess for**
      1. Possible etiologies as documented in the medical history (history of bladder or prostate cancer, neurologic disorders, recent radiation or chemotherapy)
      2. Signs and symptoms of urinary tract infection
      3. Indwelling catheter function, assess catheter and balloon size as possible source of spasm
      4. Hematuria
      5. Food and fluid intake: some foods aggravate symptoms; adequate fluid intake important for urinary tract health
      6. Presence of fecal impaction

   D. **Potential Diagnoses**
      1. Pain related to bladder spasm secondary to obstruction/infection/disease process
      2. Altered urinary elimination related to bladder spasm
      3. Patient and family knowledge deficit related to disease process, management of indwelling catheter, and treatment of bladder spasm

E. **Planning and Intervention: etiology will guide treatment**
   1. Presence of indwelling catheter
      a) Reassess the need for Foley catheter
      b) Change catheter to appropriate size
      c) Partially deflate balloon
      d) Gently irrigate with normal saline
      e) May need to initiate continuous saline irrigation if etiology is related to blood clots
   2. Urinary tract infection
      a) Antibiotics
      b) Reassess the need for Foley catheter
      c) Change catheter if catheterized
      d) Increase oral fluid intake if feasible
   3. Disimpact if etiology is fecal impaction
   4. Non-pharmacologic measures: assisting the patient to void every 4 hours, sitting or standing to void, teach relaxation techniques
   5. Pharmacologic measures: antispasmodic drugs such as oxybutynin (Ditropan®); NSAIDs; hyoscyamine

F. **Patient and Family Education**
   1. Explain etiology of bladder spasm and measures to reduce symptoms
   2. Demonstrate proper catheter care and explain signs and symptoms of catheter obstruction
   3. Explain signs and symptoms of urinary tract infection
   4. Teach expected medication effects and potential side effects

G. **Evaluate**
   1. Effectiveness of interventions and/or medications in decreasing pain related to bladder spasm
   2. Effectiveness of antibiotic therapy, if appropriate
   3. Patient and family understanding of interventions and medication regimen and recognition of symptoms

H. **Revise plan according to findings from ongoing evaluations, changes in patient status, or family needs**

VIII. Bowel Incontinence

A. **Definition: the inability to control bowel movements**

B. **Possible Etiologies**

1. Obstruction, including fecal impaction or tumor (overflow incontinence)

2. Diarrhea (See Section XI: Diarrhea)

3. Sphincter damage due to rectal carcinoma, recto-vaginal fistula, or inflammatory bowel disease involving the rectum

4. Sensory or motor dysfunction of the rectal sphincter due to spinal cord lesions or compression, multiple sclerosis, diabetes

5. Changes in sphincter tone related to age or spinal cord compression

6. Dementia or mobility related (unable to verbalize or recognize need or unable to reach the toilet)

C. **Assess for**

1. Rectal urgency and passage of loose or formed stool without patient control; incontinence of formed stool usually related to dementia,[7] fecal impaction

2. Functional status: is patient able to reach toilet?

3. Neurologic and sensory function

4. Skin integrity

D. **Potential Diagnoses**

1. Bowel incontinence related to obstruction, diarrhea, neurosensory dysfunction, or impaired cognition

2. Risk for impaired skin integrity related to bowel incontinence

3. Patient and family knowledge deficit related to etiology and management of bowel incontinence

4. Patient and family anxiety related to bowel incontinence

E. **Planning and Intervention: etiology will guide interventions**

1. Review bowel regimen and adjust laxative dose as needed if patient is taking opioids for pain

2. Utilize opioids for constipating effect

3. Disimpact if fecal impaction is causing incontinence; may need opioid or anxiolytic prior to disimpaction

4. Modify dietary practices if appropriate and as tolerated

    a) Decrease fiber intake to reduce bulk formation of stool

    b) Increase fluid intake of lukewarm, room temperature, or cool beverages (very cold or hot liquids can act as stimulants)

    c) Avoid spicy, greasy, rich, and fried foods; avoid caffeine and high amounts of milk products

    d) Incorporate bananas, rice, applesauce into diet; eat several small frequent meals rather than large meals

5. Alter environment to place patient closer to toileting facilities
6. Initiate a bowel routine (i.e., taking patient to toilet after eating)
7. Maintain skin integrity with adequate skin cleansing and liberal use of skin protectant ointment
8. Utilize incontinence products

F. Patient and Family Education

1. Explain etiology of bowel incontinence, and appropriate interventions relative to the etiology
2. Explain effects of medication and potential side effects
3. Demonstrate correct hygiene and skin care techniques to prevent skin breakdown
4. Explain safety measures if altering environment for ease in toileting (i.e., have patient call for assistance, bowel routine, assuring clear path to bathroom)

G. Evaluate

1. Effectiveness of interventions and patient and family teaching (Are patient and family satisfied with outcome?)
2. Medication effectiveness and presence of side effects
3. Skin integrity
4. Patient safety

H. Revise plan according to findings from ongoing evaluations, changes in patient status, or family needs

IX. Bowel Obstruction

A. Definition: occlusion of the lumen of the intestine, delaying or preventing the normal passage of feces

B. Possible Etiologies

1. External compression of the lumen (i.e., tumor enlargement, metastases, adhesions, organomegaly)
2. Internal occlusion of the lumen (i.e., tumor, intussusception)
3. Ischemic or inflammatory processes (i.e., Crohn's disease, diverticulitis, peritonitis, pancreatitis, hernia)
4. Fecal blockage (severe constipation can mimic obstruction)
5. Adynamic ileus (i.e., pneumonia, metabolic/electrolyte problems)
6. Metabolic disorders (i.e., hypokalemia)
7. Drugs (i.e., diuretics can cause hypokalemia, which decreases peristalsis; opioids; chemotherapy)
8. Often more than one etiology is present when a bowel obstruction develops

C. **Assess for**

1. History: predisposition to obstruction (cancer, pancreatitis, etc.), history of bowel habits, medication usage, history of pain

2. Pain

    a) Crampy, colicky pain in the middle to upper abdomen relieved with vomiting suggests a small bowel obstruction

    b) Crampy pain in the lower abdomen that increases over time suggests a large bowel obstruction

    c) Severe, steady pain is a sign of bowel strangulation

3. Abdominal distention: present and possibly severe in obstruction of the large intestine; visible peristalsis may be present; patient may complain of constipation and bloating

4. Nausea and vomiting: moderate to severe in small bowel obstruction and can relieve pain. May develop later in obstruction of the large intestine

5. Bowel sounds: hyperactive sounds and borborygmi; hypoactive or absent sounds with adynamic ileus

6. Constipation and inability to pass flatus seen in complete obstruction

7. Diarrhea due to overflow of feces related to fecal impaction

8. Fever and chills could indicate bowel ischemia or strangulation

D. **Possible Diagnoses**

1. Pain related to bowel obstruction

2. Potential for fluid and electrolyte imbalances related to vomiting secondary to bowel obstruction

3. Anxiety related to pain and inability to defecate secondary to bowel obstruction

4. Nausea and vomiting related to bowel obstruction

5. Patient and family knowledge deficit related to etiology and treatment of bowel obstruction

E. **Planning and Intervention**

1. Disimpact if necessary, utilizing an opioid or anxiolytic if needed for patient comfort

2. Surgery may be considered if

    a) This is patient's first obstruction

    b) The obstruction occurs in only one site

    c) The patient's prognosis and condition will allow for a good outcome[8]

    d) Surgery is not usually indicated for non-mechanical obstructions

3. Medication for pain including antispasmodics (loperamide or scopolamine), and opioids

4. Stimulant laxatives (senna, bisacodyl) and prokinetics (metoclopramide) should be discontinued if patient is experiencing colicky pain or complete bowel obstruction[8]

5. Medication for nausea and vomiting (if symptoms are distressful for patient) including promethazine, prochlorperazine, or haloperidol
6. Gastric decompression using nasogastric (NG) suction may be necessary for relief of gastric distention and nausea; if symptoms persist, percutaneous gastrostomy placement can aid in venting
7. Oral fluids should be increased if tolerable and nausea and vomiting can be controlled; parenteral fluids may be considered if vomiting is not controlled and patient at risk for severe dehydration
8. Treat constipation or diarrhea according to interventions outlined in Sections X and XI

F. **Patient and Family Education**
1. Explain etiology and treatment course of bowel obstruction
2. Explain medication effects and possible side effects
3. Demonstrate post-operative care of incisions/gastrostomy tube, if appropriate
4. Explain importance of bowel regimen, and assist in initiating regimen, if appropriate

G. **Evaluate**
1. Effectiveness of interventions and patient and family teaching
2. Effects and side effects of medications
3. Patient and family understanding of treatment and prevention of further obstruction

H. **Revise plan according to findings from ongoing evaluations, changes in patient status, or family needs**

X. **Constipation**

A. **Definition: difficulty in passing stools or an incomplete or infrequent passage of hard stools**

B. **Possible Etiologies**
1. Intestinal obstruction: tumors in bowel wall, external compression of the bowel by pelvic or abdominal tumors
2. Medications: opioids, tricyclic antidepressants, phenothiazines, antacids, diuretics, iron, vincristine, anti-hypertensives, anticonvulsants, anticholinergics or drugs with anticholinergic effects, NSAIDs
3. Metabolic disorders: hypercalcemia, hypokalemia, hypothyroidism
4. Other disease processes or disorders: colitis, diverticular disease
5. Dietary problems: low fiber intake, inadequate fluid intake, dehydration
6. Neurologic: confusion, depression, sedation
7. Weakness, inactivity, and immobility
8. Pain associated with constipation, including anal fissures or hemorrhoids, straining at stool, etc.

9. Decrease in privacy or unfamiliar toilet facilities; patient reluctant to ask for help in toileting (embarrassment, loss of independence, do not want to be a burden, etc.)

C. **Assess for**

1. Bowel history

    a) Last bowel movement and bowel movement prior to last

    (1) Ask if the last bowel movement was full and satisfying

    b) Amount, color, consistency

    c) Straining or pain during defecation

    d) Current bowel regimen: does patient need aids in defecation, such as laxatives, suppositories, or digital removal

2. Food and fluid intake

3. Mobility potential

4. Abdominal assessment: abdominal distension and/or tenderness; may report feeling of fullness or bloating; bowel sounds may be normal or hypoactive; percussion reveals dullness in otherwise tympanic areas; may be able to palpate stool in colon

5. Increase in flatus

6. Nausea, vomiting

7. Rectal examination: presence of hemorrhoids, anal fissures; digital examination might reveal hard stool or large amount of soft stool in rectum

8. Patient and family understanding of underlying cause of constipation, expected effects of medication or non-pharmacologic remedies

D. **Potential Diagnoses**

1. Risk for constipation related to opioid or other constipating medication usage, immobility, decrease in food, fluid intake

2. Constipation related to opioid medication usage, immobility, decrease in food, fluid intake

3. Alteration in comfort related to constipation

4. Patient and family knowledge deficit related to appropriate bowel regimen

E. **Planning and Intervention**

1. Goal in control of opioid-induced constipation is prevention of constipation

2. Bowel obstruction should be ruled out and disimpaction considered if appropriate

    a) If digitally disimpacting, give an opioid or anxiolytic prior to intervention

    b) Digital disimpaction contraindicated in neutropenic or thrombocytopenic patients; may be contraindicated in end stage cardiac patients

3. Non-pharmacologic therapies

    a) Increase fluid intake: water and fruit juices are most effective (prune juice is especially helpful)

- b) Encourage high-fiber foods; examples include: whole grain breads and cereals, bran cereal, fresh, canned, frozen or dried fruits, and vegetables
- c) Increase activity, including active or passive range of motion if possible
- d) Ask patient what has been effective in the past

4. Pharmacologic therapies
    - a) If patient is at risk for constipation, including those on opioids, prophylactic stool softener and stimulant laxatives should be started (example: Peri-Colace® or senna with docusate sodium)[9]
    - b) Patient may use own regimen, but regular use should be stressed, especially if using opioids
    - c) If no bowel movement in three days, regardless of intake, fluids should be increased if possible and an osmotic laxative (i.e., lactulose, sorbitol) started
    - d) For continuing constipation, a glycerin or bisacodyl suppository or sodium biphosphate enema may be added[9]
    - e) Discontinue medications that may cause constipation if not medically necessary (i.e., iron or calcium supplements)

5. Rectal pain or discomfort: consider hemorrhoid preparations or warm sitz baths (rule out herpes in the case of a patient with HIV disease)

F. Patient and Family Education

1. Explain etiology of constipation and instruct in ways to manage
    - a) Non-pharmacological interventions: increased food/fluid intake, increase activity
    - b) Pharmacological interventions
2. Continually reinforce necessity of bowel regime, even if patient is not constipated
3. Explain medication effects and possible side effects
4. Reinforce that bowel movement should occur at least every three days, and further action should be taken if no bowel movement after this time

G. Evaluate

1. Effectiveness of bowel regime
    - a) How often is patient having bowel movement?
    - b) Is patient having difficulty during passage of stool?
2. Assess abdomen and rectum (externally and digitally, if appropriate)
3. Patient and family understanding of bowel regime, including medications and non-pharmacologic measures to prevent constipation

H. Revise plan according to findings from ongoing evaluations, changes in patient status, or family needs

XI. Diarrhea

A. Definition: the frequent passage of loose, unformed, liquid stool

B. Possible Etiologies

1. Laxative therapy overuse or imbalance
2. Side effect of other drugs (i.e., NSAIDs, antibiotics)
3. Radiation and chemotherapy
4. Food intolerances or tube feedings
5. Malnutrition (cachexia related to cancer or AIDS)
6. Surgical procedures: gastrectomy, ileal resection, colectomy
7. Fecal impaction
8. Infection (especially as seen in immunocompromised patients, such as those with AIDS and post-chemotherapy)
9. Partial intestinal obstruction
10. Tumors: gastrointestinal and carcinoid tumors, pancreatic islet cell tumors, small cell lung tumors
11. Gastrointestinal disorders: inflammatory bowel disease, pancreatic insufficiency, diverticulitis, ulcerative colitis, Crohn's disease
12. Other chronic disorders such as diabetes and hyperthyroidism

C. Assessment

1. History, including characteristic of stool, how often stool is occurring, medication usage, recent radiation or chemotherapy treatments, or gastrointestinal surgery
2. Physical exam
    a) Abdominal assessment: bowel sounds may be hyperactive (or hypoactive to absent if intestinal obstruction is present), patient reports of cramping or pain, palpable masses in abdomen may indicate partial obstruction
    b) Nature and consistency of stool (if available to assess): pancreatic insufficiency is indicated by steatorrhea (loose, pale, foul-smelling, greasy stool); fecal impaction may be indicated by small amounts of loose stool
3. Signs of dehydration
4. Skin integrity

D. Potential Diagnoses

1. Diarrhea related to infection, metabolic disorders, medications or therapies, partial obstruction, malnutrition, or gastrointestinal intolerance to food/feedings
2. Risk for impaired skin integrity related to diarrhea

3. Potential for fluid and electrolyte imbalance related to diarrhea
4. Patient and family knowledge deficit related to etiology and treatment of diarrhea

E. **Planning and Intervention: etiology will guide treatment options**
   1. Increase fluid intake, preferably with electrolyte replacement drinks
   2. Clear liquid diet for first 24 hours, with light carbohydrates (rice, crackers, etc.), then advance as tolerated to diet high in protein and calories; avoid spicy, greasy, high-fiber foods and foods high in lactose or caffeine; small, frequent meals are usually better tolerated. Incorporate bananas, rice, applesauce into diet to help keep stool firm in consistency
   3. Disimpact if necessary, utilizing opioids or anxiolytics prior to intervention, if needed for patient comfort
   4. Discontinue laxatives if certain etiology of diarrhea is not due to impaction
   5. Antidiarrheals: loperamide; diphenoxylate HCl with atropine (adsorbent agents do not work as fast, so are not indicated in advanced disease); opioids can also be considered if patient is not already taking
   6. Pancreatic insufficiency: pancreatic enzymes with meals, with loperamide (slows peristalsis)
   7. Maintain skin integrity with adequate skin cleansing and liberal use of skin protectant ointment

F. **Patient and Family Education**
   1. Explain etiology of diarrhea, and appropriate interventions relative to the etiology
   2. Explain effects of medication and potential side effects
   3. Demonstrate correct hygiene and skin care techniques to prevent skin breakdown
   4. Explain signs, symptoms, and treatment of dehydration

G. **Evaluate**
   1. Effectiveness of interventions and patient and family teaching (Are patient and family satisfied with outcome?)
   2. Medication effectiveness and presence of side effects
   3. Skin integrity
   4. Fluid volume status

H. **Revise plan according to findings from ongoing evaluations, changes in patient status, or family needs**

XII. Dysphagia/Odynophagia

A. **Dysphagia: a subjective awareness of difficulty in swallowing**

1. Possible etiologies[2]

   a) Obstructive: cancer of esophagus and other cancers of the head and neck area, benign peptic stricture and lower esophageal ring; gastroesophageal reflux disease (GERD), compression of vessels or mediastinal nodes. This type of dysphagia is intermittent, usually occurring when eating or drinking; solid foods are most difficult foods to swallow; some patients can tolerate only liquids

   b) Motor: neuromuscular, esophageal dysfunction (stasis) related to smooth muscle hypertonia or dystonia: e.g., cardiospasm, esophageal aperistalsis, diffuse esophageal spasm (GERD), amyotrophic lateral sclerosis, Parkinson's disease, multiple sclerosis and dementia; this type of dysphagia is often for both solids and liquids

   c) Systemic dysphagia: scleroderma, inflammation and infections affect swallowing ability

   d) General deconditioning: chronic diseases can cause fatigue and general deconditioning

      (1) Medications that can contribute to dysphagia include anticholinergics, tricyclic antidepressants, antipsychotics and neuroleptic medications by causing dryness, slowing esophageal peristalsis and decreasing swallowing coordination

B. **Odynophagia: a report of painful swallowing**

1. Odynophagia possible etiologies

   a) Inflammatory process: candidiasis, conditions favoring overgrowth of fungal *Candida albicans* (e.g., broad spectrum antibiotics, diabetes mellitus, compromised cellular immunity—AIDS, leukemia, chemotherapy)

   b) Dry mucous membranes due to xerostomia (decreased quantity or quality of saliva) from radiotherapy, anticholinergic or other medications

   c) Corrosive esophagitis (ingestion of substance damaging to mucosa)

   d) Bronchoesophageal fistula with chief complaint: "coughing after ingesting fluids"

C. **Assess for**

1. Etiology of dysphagia or odynophagia, which will direct intervention plan

2. If odynophagia only, treatment of underlying cause may relieve symptom

   a) Assess oral cavity including tongue, gingiva, mucosa, lips, presence and amount of saliva

   b) Note onset and duration of painful swallowing

   c) Assess voice quality, swallowing ability, oral hygiene

   d) Oral intake: review 24 hour quantity food/liquid

   e) Review history for AIDS, diabetes, chemotherapy, radiotherapy

   f) Review current medications for contributing agents (steroid inhalers, steroids, antibiotics, sulfa)

g) Presence of creamy white curd-like patches in oropharynx, tongue; patches usually scrape off easily with 4x4 gauze; may cause bleeding

3. Current nutritional status related to disease process, goals of therapies, patient and family expectations

4. If dysphagia, odynophagia are accompanied by anorexia, evaluate patient for disease progression, current nutritional status; discuss management options with interdisciplinary team, patient and family

D. Potential Diagnoses

1. Swallowing impairment, nutritional impairment related to dysphagia (amount of time) or odynophagia (amount of time)

2. Oral mucous membranes impairment related to: candidiasis, mucositis, xerostomia

3. Patient and family knowledge deficit of: nutrition; types of food, liquids; safety in food selection, expected medication, therapy effects and side effects

E. Planning and Intervention

1. If candidiasis: antifungal swish and swallow QID for 7–10 days; OR antifungal PO for 5–7 days

2. If mucositis or esophagitis from radiotherapy: topical anesthetic, antihistamine, antacid combination (e.g., lidocaine/diphenhydrAMINE/antacid in 1:1:1 ratio as swish and swallow IF patient has gag reflex)

3. If obstruction from tumors/nodes: limited dose steroids may reduce inflammatory edema

4. If neuro-motor etiology: speech therapy consult may be helpful to evaluate swallow and make recommendation

5. If dry mucosa induced from medications or radiotherapy: artificial saliva, lip balm, exquisite oral care, increase hydration

6. Determine food consistency best tolerated by patient: liquids may have thickening agents added to facilitate swallowing

7. If medications are etiology of dysphagia or odynophagia, consider alternative medicines if appropriate

8. Artificial feeding may be considered for obstructive or fistula processes in some palliative care situations depending upon the patient's place on the disease trajectory, current nutritional and functional status and other factors

F. Patient and Family Education

1. Importance of excellent oral hygiene

2. Avoid nicotine, alcohol and caffeine, which increase esophageal and vasospasm and have mucosal drying effects

3. Cool, non-irritating foods and liquids generally better tolerated

4. Encourage patient to chew food well and to avoid large boluses of meat, bread; modify food consistency if necessary (e.g., ground or pureed meats)

5. Anticipated medication effects and potential side effects

G. **Evaluate for effectiveness of interventions, specifically**

1. Resolution of candidiasis
2. Improvement in mucosal lubrication
3. Oral hygiene
4. Nutritional status
5. Patient and family understanding of instructions, recommendations

H. **Revise plan according to findings from ongoing evaluations, changes in patient status, or family needs**

XIII. Dyspnea/Cough

A. **Definitions**

1. Dyspnea: subjective sensation of shortness of breath
2. Cough: a natural defense of the body to prevent entry of foreign material into the respiratory tract[10]

B. **Possible Etiologies**

1. Dyspnea: lung tumor or metastases, pleural effusion, COPD, CHF, ascites, pneumothorax, pulmonary embolism, anemia, neurologic insult
2. Cough: infection, inflammation, cardiac (left ventricular failure), pulmonary disease (pleural effusion, bronchospasm, bronchogenic cancer), medications (ACE inhibitors), smoke, tobacco abuse or irritation from second-hand smoke, allergic conditions, GERD

C. **Assess for**

1. Dyspnea: etiology will direct intervention plan

    a) Onset of dyspnea, respiratory rate, depth, quality of respiration, lung sounds, accessory muscle use, stridor

    b) Past interventions that have provided relief/comfort

    c) Appropriate use and understanding of current medications for relief of dyspnea and accompanying anxiety

    d) Whether patient is a carbon dioxide (CO_2) retainer; this will influence decisions regarding oxygen delivery rate, opioid and anxiolytic dosing

    e) Patient and family anxiety, coping, understanding of dyspnea triggers and etiology, and interventions to control dyspnea

2. Cough: etiology will direct intervention plan

   a) History and physical to determine etiology and appropriate treatment

      (1) Productive vs. nonproductive cough

      (2) If productive, sputum quantity and appearance

      (3) Diagnostic studies as appropriate

   b) Effect of cough on patient and family's quality of life

   c) Need for cough suppressant OR cough expectorant based on etiology and patient need

D. **Potential Diagnoses**

   1. Respiratory alteration related to: impairment of airway clearance, breathing pattern, or gas exchange

   2. Patient and family knowledge deficit of: etiology or triggers of dyspnea and/or cough, steps to relieve dyspnea or anxiety; medication use, effects or side effects

   3. Patient discomfort related to inability to control cough and/or mobilize secretions

   4. Patient and family anxiety related to perceived situational powerlessness, fear, breathing impairment

E. **Planning and Intervention**[10]

   1. Review of medical history, progression of disease, current medications; etiology of dyspnea will direct intervention plan

   2. Non-pharmacologic interventions

      a) Dyspnea

         (1) Position patient in high Fowler's position as appropriate; COPD patients do better leaning forward with upper arms supported on a table

         (2) Encourage pursed lip breathing in COPD patients

         (3) Palliative thoracentesis or paracentesis may be considered in selected patients

         (4) Model calm reassurance

         (5) Encourage intake of nutrient-dense beverages (e.g., commercial supplements) if oral intake is limited because of dyspnea; liquids take less eating effort

         (6) Fan directly in front of patient; cool room environment

         (7) Complementary therapies such as relaxation techniques, guided imagery, therapeutic touch

         (8) Oxygen as appropriate

      b) Productive cough: chest physiotherapy (if able to tolerate), oxygen, humidity and suctioning, elevate head of bed, frequent sips of water, throat lozenges

3. Pharmacologic interventions

   a) Dyspnea and productive cough

      (1) Opioids (PO, SL, SQ, IV or nebulized) for bronchodilatation

         i. Start low (e.g., 5 mg PO every 2 hours, PRN) and titrate dose slowly for opioid-naïve patients and patients with CO_2 retention

         ii. Monitor respiratory rate and depth

      (2) High dose steroids for obstructive or inflammatory etiologies

      (3) Antibiotics for infection if appropriate

      (4) Anxiolytic medications may help to reduce the anxiety that often accompanies dyspnea: use and titrate slowly in elderly, dementia patients and patients with CO_2 retention; monitor respiratory rate and depth

      (5) For uncontrolled dyspnea in hospice home-care setting, may consider short-term inpatient management

      (6) Sedation at end of life for refractory dyspnea is an option

   b) Nonproductive cough: non-opioid (dextromethorphan, benzonatate) or opioid antitussives, inhaled anesthetic (lidocaine, bupivacaine)

      (1) Nebulized lidocaine (e.g., 1%–5 ml) for 10 minutes every 2–6 hours

      (2) NPO for 1 hour post treatment due to risk of aspiration from loss of gag reflex from anesthetic agent

F. **Patient and Family Education**

   1. Reassurance and empowerment of patient and family by review, rehearsal of steps to take when patient's shortness of breath begins

   2. Treatment options, medication effects, side effects

   3. Demonstrate relaxation techniques when patient and family is not in crisis

   4. Instruct others not to crowd dyspneic person and to remain calm, in control of emotions

   5. Consistency in information with rehearsal, review by all members of the interdisciplinary team

G. **Evaluate**

   1. Understanding, compliance and effectiveness of medications for dyspneic episodes

   2. For patient and family coping; reduction of, improvement in management and control of dyspneic episodes

   3. For progression of disease process related to uncontrolled dyspnea

H. **Revise plan according to findings from ongoing evaluations, changes in patient status, or family needs**

XIV. Edema

A. Definition: presence of excessive fluid in the intercellular tissues especially in the subcutaneous tissues

B. Possible Etiologies

1. Protein deficiency
2. Obstruction of venous return: peritoneal tumors, DVT, CHF, superior vena cava syndrome (SVC)
3. Renal failure
4. Lymphedema: blockage of lymphatic return in the periphery or the abdomen from surgical procedures, pressure from tumor
5. Ascites of liver failure; peritoneal inflammation

C. Assess for

1. Review of medical history and progression of disease process
2. Etiology of edema, which will direct intervention plan
3. New, increased or returning edema
4. Extremity edema, pitting, non-pitting, tissue perfusion, warmth, cold, presence or absence of leaking from tissues
5. Superior vena cava syndrome (SVC)
    a) Upper body edema (i.e., papilledema, facial edema, distended neck veins, one or both arms depending on where the obstruction is located); note onset, tissues involved
    b) Other symptoms: dyspnea (most common), headache, chest pain, dry cough, visual or mental status changes, dizziness, vertigo
    c) SVC is considered an oncologic emergency and may be palliated with radiotherapy with or without steroids depending on the etiology
    d) Not responsive to diuretics
6. Ascites: abdomen size, tenderness, distention, fluid wave; if elevated diaphragm, may have dyspnea, pleural effusion
7. Patient and family understanding of disease process related to poor perfusion, expected medication effects and possible side effects

D. Potential Diagnoses

1. Tissue perfusion alteration related to: peripheral edema, ascites, upper body, head and neck edema
2. Skin integrity impairment and risk related to poor perfusion, subcutaneous tissue edema, increased pressure points

3. Respiratory alteration related to gas exchange impairment (for dyspnea related to ascites, SVC syndrome)

4. Patient and family knowledge deficit of disease process, expected medication effects or possible side effects, non-pharmacologic measures

E. **Planning and Intervention**

1. Etiology of edema will direct intervention plan

2. Symptomatic relief of ascites: spironolactone, paracentesis; the success of the diuretics in reducing ascites depends on the cause of the ascites[11]

3. Symptomatic relief of peripheral edema: compression stockings; diuretics usually appropriate when there are also crackles heard in lungs; meticulous skin care; active or passive exercise to help venous return if patient can tolerate; limb elevation above level of heart

4. Lymphedema

   a) Does not respond to diuretics unless there is a true peripheral edema component

   b) May not resolve despite elevation, compression stockings

   c) In the palliative care patient not actively dying, manual lymph drainage therapies may promote better quality of life

F. **Patient and Family Education**

1. Explain etiology of edema and instruct in ways to manage or reduce

2. Expected medication effects and possible side effects

3. Application of compression stockings prior to ambulation

4. Post-paracentesis care

G. **Evaluate**

1. Effectiveness of medication

2. For level, return, extension of edema

3. Patient and family understanding of disease process, medications, application and use of compression stockings and/or manual lymph drainage therapies; non-pharmacologic interventions

H. **Revise plan according to findings from ongoing evaluations, changes in patient status, or family needs**

XV. **Extrapyramidal Symptoms (EPS)**

A. **Definition: involuntary movements, hyperkinetic (akathisia) or hypokinetic (dystonia); tardive dyskinesia is a late-effect, which may not respond to reversal therapies**

B. **Possible Etiologies**
   1. Iatrogenic drug-induced from
      a) Neuroleptics
      b) Phenothiazines (e.g., chlorpromazine)
      c) Butyrophenones (e.g., haloperidol)
      d) Clozapine
      e) Metoclopramide
      f) Opioids (myoclonus)
   2. Parkinson's disease, chorea
   3. Cerebral lesions

C. **Assess for**
   1. Etiology of EPS from medical history, medication review which will direct intervention plan
   2. Possible iatrogenic response to a medical therapy used to treat a symptom
   3. Patient safety with ambulation, activities of daily living (ADLs)
   4. Patient and family anxiety relating to EPS, understanding of medication effects and side effects

D. **Diagnosis**
   1. Impaired physical mobility related to neurologic impairment caused by etiology
   2. Self-care deficit related to immobility, hyperactivity, loss of coordination
   3. Patient and family knowledge deficit related to medication effects or side effects, safety needs

E. **Planning and Intervention**
   1. For phenothiazine toxicity
      a) Stop phenothiazine
      b) Benztropine mesylate (Cogentin®), trihexyphenidyl, or diphenhydrAMINE
   2. For akathisia (inability to sit still, pacing, agitation, restless movements)
      a) Benzodiazepines (lorazepam, diazepam)
      b) Beta-blockers (propranolol)
   3. For dystonia, slow, retarded movements: physical or occupational therapy may be an adjunct if appropriate according to patient's place in the disease process, trajectory
   4. In elderly, or others who may have sensitivity to anticholinergics: amantadine
   5. Review of symptoms being treated with medication that may cause EPS; if symptoms remain present, discussion with medical team regarding alternative medications to control

F. **Patient and Family Education**

1. Stopping medication that may be contributing to EPS
2. Expected medication effects and potential side effects
3. Monitoring patient activity; safety in ambulation

G. **Evaluate for effectiveness of interventions, specifically**

1. Effect of medication change on EPS symptoms
2. Patient and family compliance, comfort with new medications
3. Control of symptoms

H. **Revise plan according to findings from ongoing evaluations, changes in patient status, or family needs**

XVI. Hematologic Symptoms

A. **Definitions**

1. Hemorrhage: excessive bleeding
2. Clotting: systemic response to disease or medication that initiates coagulation cascade causing clotting
3. Cytopenia: reduction in bone marrow blood cell components, which can precipitate a systemic response

   a) Neutropenia: reduction in white blood cells; decreases patient's ability to respond to infection

   b) Thrombocytopenia: reduction in platelets; increases potential for frank, uncontrolled bleeding

   c) Anemias: reduction in production or maturation of red blood cells; low hemoglobin; decreased oxygen carrying cells; increased dyspnea, fatigue

   d) Pancytopenia: reduction in all blood cells

B. **Possible Etiologies**

1. Initiating coagulation cascade: deep vein thrombosis (DVT)
2. Immunologic processes (AIDS), drug-induced processes, prosthetic cardiac valves, veno-occlusive liver disease initiating coagulation cascade: hemorrhage, disseminated intravascular coagulopathy (DIC)
3. Chemotherapy, radiotherapy or disorders of spleen: thrombocytopenia, pancytopenia
4. Tumor erosion of blood vessels: hemorrhage
5. Pulmonary embolism (PE)

C. Assess for

1. Review medical history and current medications for potential hematology problems
2. Review current medications, foods, herbals for interactions with anticoagulant therapy
3. For DIC: petechiae, ecchymosis, oozing blood from mucous membranes, body orifices, puncture sites, signs of decreased perfusion to brain, kidneys, gastrointestinal, cardiovascular and peripheral vascular systems, lungs
4. For DVT: possible peripheral phlebitis, noting vascular access devices, streaking, erythema, heat over vein
5. For pulmonary embolism: sudden onset dyspnea
6. For thrombocytopenia: periorbital petechiae, epistaxis, gingival bleeding, blood-streaked sputum, emesis, urine or stool; acute shortness of breath, inspiratory pain, vaginal bleeding, petechiae, ecchymosis, joint pain, change in mental status, paresthesias
7. Patient and family understanding of and coping with changes in blood clotting response or pancytopenia; non-pharmacologic therapies, safety

D. Potential Diagnoses

1. Injury risk due to altered clotting patterns related to etiology
2. Infection risk due to neutropenia and body's reduced ability to control or fight infection
3. Patient and family knowledge deficit related to expected medication effects or side effects, safety needs, e.g., injury or infection
4. Medication risk related to anticoagulant therapy and other medications, herbals, foods

E. Plan and Intervention: treat underlying problem if appropriate

1. For DVT: anticoagulant therapy; monitor for other medications, foods and herbals that may interfere with anticoagulant therapy; anti-embolic stockings
2. For PE: anticoagulant therapy; monitor other medications, food and herbals that may interfere with anticoagulant therapy; anti-embolic stockings, treatment of dyspnea, pain
3. For thrombocytopenia
   a) If palliative care: bleeding precautions, platelet transfusion for platelets <10,000, if appropriate
   b) If hospice: bleeding precautions, treat bleeding with compression, other non-pharmacologic interventions
4. For DIC: replenish clotting factors, e.g., platelets, fresh frozen plasma, antithrombin factor in palliative care; patient should be in an acute care facility for ongoing monitoring during therapy
5. For neutropenia: institute precautions against introduction of bacteria, infections to patient
6. Patient and family support, instruction, reassurance during bleeding and in anticipation of bleed

F. **Patient and Family Education**

1. Bleeding precautions

    a) Soft toothbrush and gentle motions for tooth brushing

    b) Care when using eating utensils

    c) Rinses for mouth

    d) No suppositories

    e) Safety in ambulation; prevent falls, injury

    f) Use electric razor rather than straight razor

2. For active bleed: long pressure for active bleed; use of dark towels; whom to call

3. For PE: elevate head of bed for dyspnea; palliative oxygen if needed

4. For DVT: use of anti-embolic stockings applied before ambulation; expected anticoagulation medicine effects and side effects

5. Medicines, food, and herbals that can affect anticoagulation including vitamin E (greater than 1000–1500 units/day), theophylline, carbamazepine, phenytoin, vitamin K (especially high in dark green vegetables)

6. For neutropenia: regular and frequent hand washing; plants, flowers not in direct proximity; support of family in encouraging visitors with colds, illness to visit when they are well

7. Review, rehearse with patient and family the steps to take if bleeding begins

G. **Evaluate**

1. Effectiveness of medical therapies

2. Patient compliance with anticoagulant therapy; for therapeutic PTT (partial thromboplastin time), PT (prothrombin time), INR (international normalized ratio)

3. Safety in ambulation

4. Patient and family understanding regarding disease process, safety, expected medicine effects, and potential side effects

H. **Revise plan according to findings from ongoing evaluations, changes in patient status, or family needs**

XVII. **Hiccoughs**

A. **Definition: an involuntary contraction of the diaphragm, followed by rapid closure of the glottis**

B. **Possible Etiologies**

1. Gastric distention: impaired gastric motility, excessive gas

2. Central nervous system: neoplasm, stroke, multiple sclerosis, ventriculoperitoneal shunts, arteriovenous malformations, hydrocephalus, lesions from head trauma

3. Peripheral nervous system: irritation of phrenic or vagus nerve
4. Tumors of the neck, lung, mediastinum
5. Chest surgery or trauma
6. Respiratory disorders: pulmonary edema, pneumonia, bronchitis, asthma, COPD
7. Gastrointestinal disorders: esophagitis or esophageal obstruction, gastritis, peptic ulcer disease, gastric cancer, pancreatitis, pancreatic cancer, bowel obstruction, cholelithiasis/cholecystitis
8. Renal/hepatic disorders
9. Metabolic disorders: uremia, hypocalcemia, hyponatremia
10. Infectious disease: sepsis, influenza, herpes zoster, malaria, tuberculosis
11. Pharmacologic agents: general anesthesia, IV corticosteroids, barbiturates, benzodiazepines, diazepam, chlordiazepoxide
12. Psychogenic: stress, excitement, grief reactions, anorexia, personality disorders

C. Assess for

1. Etiology of hiccoughs related to medical/psychological history and/or medication usage
2. Associated signs and symptoms (underlying disease process, etc.)
3. Severity and duration of current episode and previous episodes
4. Relationship of hiccoughs to sleep: hiccoughs that stop during sleep suggest a psychogenic cause
5. Patient and family concerns and knowledge: Are the hiccoughs troublesome? Does anything help to alleviate hiccoughs?

D. Diagnoses

1. Alteration in comfort related to hiccoughs
2. Risk for fluid/nutritional deficit related to dysphagia secondary to hiccoughs
3. Risk for sleep pattern disturbance related to hiccoups
4. Patient and family knowledge deficit related to etiology and treatment of hiccoughs

E. Planning and Intervention: etiology of hiccoughs can guide intervention plan (i.e., possible reversal of metabolic disorders)

1. Non-pharmacologic interventions: before suggesting non-pharmacologic techniques, assure patient safety and do not suggest techniques that may be harmful, depending upon diagnosis

   a) Nasopharyngeal stimulation
      (1) Swallowing one teaspoon of granulated sugar
      (2) Lifting uvula with a spoon or cotton-tip applicator
      (3) Gargling with water

- (4) Biting on a lemon
- (5) Swallowing crushed ice

b) Interference with normal respiratory function
- (1) Induction of sneezing or coughing
- (2) Re-breathing into paper bag
- (3) Breath holding or hyperventilation

c) Etiology related to gastric distention
- (1) Nasogastric suction
- (2) Gastric lavage

d) Complementary therapies
- (1) Hypnosis and/or behavior modification
- (2) Acupuncture

e) Distraction

2. Pharmacologic therapies

a) If etiology is related to gastric distention
- (1) Simethicone before or after meals
- (2) Metoclopramide alone or with simethicone before meals

b) Peppermint oil relaxes lower esophageal sphincter and is useful for hiccoughs related to esophageal disorders; has opposing action with metoclopramide
- (1) Do not use peppermint oil for patients with GERD

c) Baclofen (5–10 mg PO TID, PRN) if simethicone and metoclopramide fail

d) Calcium channel blockers (e.g., NIFEdipine)

e) Chlorpromazine 25–50 mg TID effective for uremic etiology, but useful in other etiologies as well; postural hypotension a significant side effect, especially when used IV

f) Anticonvulsants: carbamazepine, phenytoin, and valproic acid

g) Nebulized lidocaine (3 ml of injectable 2% nebulized lidocaine in a standard small-particle nebulizer)

3. Invasive techniques

a) Phrenic nerve interruption with bupivacaine or surgery

b) Pacing electrodes for direct phrenic nerve or diaphragmatic stimulation

F. **Patient and Family Education**

1. Explain etiology and instruct in ways to treat

2. Explain appropriate, safe non-pharmacological techniques that are realistic for individual patient

3. Expected medication effects and side effects

4. Post-surgical care, if indicated

G. **Evaluate**

1. Effectiveness of non-pharmacological techniques and/or medication

2. Control of hiccoughs

3. Patient and family understanding of regimen

H. **Revise plan according to findings from ongoing evaluations, changes in patient status, or family needs**

XVIII. Impaired Mobility, Fatigue, Lethargy, Weakness

A. **Definitions**

1. Impaired mobility: a loss or abnormality of function due to physiological, anatomical, psychological or fatigue factors

2. Fatigue: a subjective sense of exhaustion with decreased motivation, ability to do activities and a decreased capacity for physical or mental activity[12]

3. Lethargy: advanced fatigue

4. Weakness: a subjective term to indicate a lack of strength as compared to what patient feels is normal

B. **Potential Etiologies**

1. Disease process

    a) Sudden onset of weakness or impaired mobility: consider neurologic deficit (e.g., spinal cord compression or other CNS tumor effects); sudden generalized weakness may be adrenal failure or septicemia

    b) Chronic disease: chronic obstructive pulmonary disease (COPD), congestive heart failure (CHF)

    c) Tumor infiltration of bone marrow

    d) Liver disease with coagulopathy

    e) Hypothyroidism: adrenal or hormonal insufficiencies (including chemical and hormonal response to tumor)

    f) Uremia: related to kidney failure, tumor, or use of nephrotoxic drugs

    g) Metabolic: hypercalcemia from metastatic disease, parathyroid disease

2. Uncontrolled pain or other symptoms, anemia, blood loss

3. Some medications or therapies may contribute to lethargy, weakness: beta blockers, antihistamines, benzodiazepines, phenothiazines, zidovudine (AZT®), myelosuppressive chemotherapy, radiation therapy

4. Nutritional deficiencies
    a) Decreased iron, B-12, folate
    b) Anorexia, nausea, vomiting, weight loss
    c) Gastrointestinal malabsorption

5. Infectious processes
    a) AIDS-related infections
    b) Pneumonia
    c) Urinary tract infections

6. Emotional factors: depression, anxiety, sleep disturbance, psychological or spiritual distress, family distress

7. Environmental factors: multiple sensory stimuli (noise, lights, odors)

C. **Assess for etiology, which will determine intervention plan**
    1. Thorough history
        a) Onset, history of or change in functional status
        b) Patient's own description of fatigue, weakness: does it relate to activity? Is it constant? Intermittent?
        c) Effect of fatigue, weakness and lethargy on quality of life using a number scale of 1 (no fatigue) to 10 (extreme fatigue)[12]
        d) Patient's place on disease trajectory of end stage or terminal illness
    2. Symptom management: review adequacy of pain control and management of other debilitating symptoms (including nausea, vomiting, dyspnea, anxiety, depression)
    3. Current medications for appropriate use and dose for patient's current weight
    4. Psychosocial factors
        a) Sleep, rest disturbance
        b) Depression, anxiety component
        c) Unresolved psychological or spiritual issues or distress
    5. Family, caregiver perceptions and impact of patient's fatigue; understanding of disease process
    6. Infectious or disease process
    7. Dyspnea if anemic

D. **Potential Diagnoses**

1. Activity alteration from fatigue due to (etiology)
2. Self-care deficit related to activity intolerance
3. Risk for altered nutritional, functional status due to activity disturbance
4. Patient and family knowledge deficit of non-pharmacologic interventions, expected medication effects, side effects
5. Impaired physical mobility related to (injury, potential for injury, pain)
6. Alteration in perceived quality of life from fatigue
7. Altered self-image and role disturbance related to change in functional abilities and endurance

E. **Planning and Interventions: etiology of fatigue, impaired mobility, lethargy, and weakness will determine intervention plan**

1. Patient's place on disease trajectory for end stage or terminal illness, wishes, and advance directives will influence treatment decisions
2. Treat specific underlying causes as appropriate
   a) If anemia: based on classification of anemia, consider treatment of cause
   b) If endocrine disorder: determine appropriate therapy
   c) If medication-induced (iatrogenic)
      (1) Consider tapering or discontinuing medicine
      (2) If opioid induced, fatigue may resolve when patient develops tolerance (usually 48–72 hours after dose increase)
      (3) If opioid induced lethargy continues and other etiologies have been ruled out and is unacceptable to the patient and family, consider adding methylphenidate 5 mg PO in the morning and at noon to combat sedation and to improve appetite and mood.[13] Titrate if not effective
3. Non-pharmacologic interventions
   a) Balance activities with rest
   b) Hospital bed and other equipment as needed to decrease fatigue from exertion
   c) Set realistic goals for ADLs and other activities
   d) Exercise, physical and occupational therapy as indicated, if tolerated
   e) Increase team services for personal care as needed

F. **Patient and Family Education**

1. Instruct regarding balancing activities and rest
2. Set activity priorities (e.g., a bedside commode may help patient to conserve the energy used walking to the bathroom for other activities)

3. Expected medication effects and potential side effects especially as they may contribute to fatigue or sedation

4. Educate family of hospice patient in terminal phase regarding end stage disease process and encourage setting of realistic expectations

5. For the palliative care patient who is not in terminal phase of disease process, discourage prolonged bedrest or excessive inactivity explaining possible adverse physical (deep vein thrombosis [DVT], pulmonary embolism [PE], pneumonia, increased weakness) and emotional (depression, decreased motivation, social isolation) effects

G. **Evaluate**

1. Effectiveness of interventions and ability of the caregivers to provide care
2. Improvement in activity tolerance
3. Patient for signs of disease progression
4. Patient and family understanding, coping with ongoing fatigue, balancing activities, prioritizing to accomplish essential or preferred activities
5. Further adjustments in team visit frequency to assist in personal care as needed

H. **Revise plan according to findings from ongoing evaluations, changes in patient status, or family needs**

XIX. **Increased Intracranial Pressure (ICP)**

A. **Definition: increase in the pressure within the cranial cavity due to increased volume of fluid or mass**

B. **Possible Etiologies**

1. Space occupying tumors, metastatic lesions with surrounding edema
2. Intracranial hemorrhage
3. Inflammatory process: abscess, encephalitis, meningitis
4. Obstruction of CSF flow

C. **Assess for**

1. Sudden unanticipated changes in patient condition with signs of increased ICP: new headache, vomiting, changed respiratory pattern, decreased motor function, lethargy to altered mental status, increased restlessness, agitation, blurred vision
2. Documentation of possible etiologies of increased ICP in past medical history
3. Patient and family anxiety, ability to cope with changes in condition; knowledge and/or understanding of presenting changes, disease process, treatment options

D. **Potential Diagnoses**

1. Altered mental status due to increased ICP
2. Cerebral alteration related to increased ICP
3. Patient and family knowledge deficit related to: disease process, current symptom changes, coping strategies

E. **Planning and Interventions**

1. Treat underlying etiology if appropriate
2. Steroids to reduce edema/inflammation
3. Anticonvulsant if seizure activity
4. Palliative radiotherapy when appropriate
5. Analgesia for headache
    a) Keep in mind that opioids can mildly increase ICP due to vasodilatation effects and mild respiratory depression
    b) Tramadol should not be used in increased ICP as it may lower seizure threshold[14]
6. Non-pharmacologic measures: head of bed 45–60 degrees, darkened room, reduce external stimuli in environment, calm presence

F. **Patient and Family Education**

1. Reassurance and instruction regarding possible cause for changes in patient condition
2. Review goals of therapy to reduce intracranial pressure symptoms and increase patient comfort and safety
3. Preparation for changes that may indicate advancement of disease and decline of patient condition; support of family/caregiver goals, needs
4. Consider transfer of home hospice patient to inpatient hospice facility or palliative care facility bed if management is beyond physical, emotional capacity of family or caregiver

G. **Evaluate**

1. Effectiveness of medications, patient comfort and relief, reduction of increased ICP symptoms
2. Patient and family understanding, coping, anxiety related to current symptoms, plan

H. **Revise plan according to findings from ongoing evaluations, changes in patient status, or family needs**

XX. **Myoclonus**

A. **Definition: twitching or brief spasm of a muscle or muscle group**

B. **Possible Etiologies**

1. High dose opioid therapy

2. Metabolic derangement (e.g., uremia)

3. Inflammatory or degenerative CNS diseases (e.g., Creutzfeldt-Jakob disease, subacute sclerosing panencephalitis, end stage Alzheimer's)

4. Hypercalcemia from osteoblastic activity of bone metastases

C. **Assess for**

1. Onset, duration of myoclonus and its impact on patient and patient functional status

2. Interruption of sleep, rest

3. Patient and family anxiety related to myoclonic jerking

4. Patient and family understanding of disease process, medication effects and side effects

5. Potential etiology which will direct intervention plan

    a) If opioid-induced, evaluate adjuvant use that would allow for pain to be managed using a reduced opioid dose or rotate opioids. Dose can often be decreased because of incomplete cross tolerance

    b) If hypercalcemia, evaluate patient's place on the disease trajectory

6. Patient safety if ambulatory or if bed bound due to uncontrolled muscular jerking movements

D. **Potential Diagnoses**

1. Alteration in metabolic status related to uremia, hypercalcemia, etc.

2. Alteration in functional status due to impairment of neuro-musculoskeletal system

3. Disturbance of sleep and rest pattern due to myoclonus

4. Patient and family knowledge deficit regarding medication effects, disease process, safety precautions

E. **Planning and Intervention: etiology of myoclonus will direct intervention plan**

1. Non-pharmacologic adjunct therapies including local heat, gentle massage, relaxation

2. If hypercalcemia etiology

    a) In palliative care, may consider pamidronate or zoledronic every 3–4 weeks to decrease serum calcium

    b) In hospice, supplementary hydration (IV or PO) may decrease serum calcium and relieve symptoms

3. If opioid-induced, consider adjuvant medicines for the specific type of pain (neuropathic or bone) at the most appropriate dose that may allow reduction in opioid dose or rotate opioids

4. If unable to treat underlying metabolic or degenerative disorder because of advanced stage of disease, patient and family wishes, treat symptoms with clonazepam, valproic acid

5. Occasionally muscle relaxants provide benefit
   a) Diazepam
   b) Baclofen
   c) Cyclobenzaprine
      (1) Cyclobenzaprine should be used cautiously in elderly or debilitated patients and considered a second line to baclofen
      (2) Increases side effects of other medications often taken by the elderly and has side effects that can contribute to conditions often already present such as CHF, glaucoma, etc.
6. If night cramps only, quinine sulfate at bedtime

F. **Patient and Family Education**
   1. Discuss possible etiologies and recommended interventions
   2. Expected medication effects and potential side effects
   3. Non-pharmacologic methods of intervention: heat, gentle massage, relaxation to decrease anxiety

G. **Evaluate for effectiveness of interventions, specifically**
   1. Decrease in or resolution of myoclonus
   2. Maintenance of effective pain control
   3. Patient and family understanding of instructions, recommendations
   4. Patient safety

H. **Revise plan according to findings from ongoing evaluations, changes in patient status, or family needs**

XXI. Nausea and Vomiting

A. **Definitions**
   1. Nausea is a subjectively perceived, stomach discomfort ranging from stomach awareness to the conscious recognition of the need to vomit
   2. Vomiting is the expelling of stomach contents through the mouth

B. **Possible Etiologies**[3,7,15]
   1. Fluid and electrolyte imbalances (hypercalcemia, hyponatremia, uremia, dehydration)
   2. Gastrointestinal disorders (pressure due to tumor, organomegaly; distention; ascites; esophageal, gastrointestinal, and hepatic malignancies; constipation; bowel obstruction; gastrointestinal stasis)
   3. Other physiologic disorders (oral thrush, cough, pain, high fever)
   4. Neurologic disorders (primary and metastatic CNS tumors, increased intracranial pressure)

5. Renal failure
6. Vestibular (tumors and bone metastases at skull base; motion sickness)
7. Chemical (radiation, medications such as chemotherapy, antibiotics, aspirin, iron, steroids, digoxin, expectorants, NSAIDs, opioids, theophylline)
8. Psychogenic (anxiety; anticipatory nausea and vomiting; fear)
9. Adverse response to certain foods especially high fat content
10. Adverse response to certain drugs, e.g., increase in opioids

C. **Assess for**

1. History of the onset of nausea and vomiting and concomitant symptoms, i.e., heartburn, constipation, excessive thirst and other symptoms that can indicate etiology
2. Pattern of nausea: when does nausea occur? Are there contributing factors?
3. If possible, assess vomitus for volume, color, odor, presence of blood (vomitus with fecal odor or fecal material indicates possible bowel obstruction; coffee ground emesis indicates old blood, whereas fresh blood indicates current hemorrhage)
4. Abdominal assessment: pain or cramps, bowel sounds, distention
5. Oropharynx for infection (thrush) or presence of tenacious sputum
6. Neurologic signs of increased intracranial pressure
7. Other factors that could trigger nausea response: malodorous wounds, pain, fear, anxiety

D. **Potential Diagnoses**

1. Nausea related to metabolic disorders, tumor pressure, drug therapies, neurosensory disorders, or anxiety
2. Risk for fluid volume deficit related to nausea and vomiting
3. Risk for altered nutrition due to intake less than body requirements related to inability to eat or keep food down secondary to nausea and vomiting
4. Patient and family knowledge deficit related to etiology and treatment of nausea and vomiting

E. **Planning and Intervention: etiology of nausea and vomiting may guide interventions**

1. Modify diet to decrease nausea
   a) Bland foods that patient enjoys, e.g., baked potatoes, soft fruits, yogurt, soft drinks, crackers or dry toast, clear liquids such as Popsicles®, JELL-O®, sports drinks, foods without aggressive odors or those that produce gas
   b) Cold or room temperature foods are often better tolerated than warm foods due to less odor
   c) Serve small, frequent meals
   d) Avoid fatty, greasy, spicy or very sweet foods
2. Correct reversible causes of nausea, including cough, hypercalcemia, increased intracranial pressure

3. Stop/hold suspected medication and obtain serum levels (digoxin, theophylline) as appropriate depending on patient's goal

4. Keep the patient cool; place a fan in the room or open a window to circulate air

5. Keep patient's head elevated

6. Medication regimen (see Table 3) should be prescribed according to etiology of nausea[3,16]

   a) A prokinetic agent (metoclopramide) can be used for delayed gastric emptying (do not use in bowel obstruction)

   b) Butyrophenones (i.e., haloperidol or droperidol [Inapsine®] for opioid-induced nausea); nausea related to opioid initiation generally resolves within one week

   c) An antihistamine (meclizine, dimenhyDRINATE) can be used for bowel obstruction or other visceral irritation (liver metastases, constipation, etc.), disturbances in the vestibular system (vertigo, motion sickness), pharyngeal stimulation (tenacious sputum, oral thrush), or increased intracranial pressure (which can also be treated with a glucocorticoid such as dexamethasone)

   d) Anticholinergics (scopolamine patches, hydroxyzine) are used primarily for increased intracranial pressure and vestibular disturbances

   e) Nausea related to disturbances in the chemoreceptor trigger zone (CTZ) (usually due to metabolic disorders, medications, and toxins produced from gastrointestinal tumors, infection, poisoning, etc.), can be treated by discontinuing offending medication if possible, and utilizing drugs which act on the CTZ (haloperidol, metoclopramide, phenothiazines)

   f) Nausea related to emetogenic chemotherapy can be treated with $5-HT_3$ serotonin receptor antagonists (ondansetron, granisetron)

   g) Nausea related to anxiety and fear can be treated with antihistamines or anticholinergics

7. Oral hygiene before and after meals

F. **Patient and Family Education**

   1. Explain etiology and treatment course of nausea and vomiting
   2. Explain effects of medication and possible side effects
   3. Explain non-pharmacologic measures to treat nausea and vomiting, including diet, oral hygiene, etc.

G. **Evaluate**

   1. Effectiveness of interventions and patient and family teaching (are patient and family satisfied with outcome?)
   2. Medication effectiveness and presence of side effects
   3. Patient and family understanding of treatment measures

H. **Revise plan according to findings from ongoing evaluations, changes in patient status, or family need**

Table 3: Management of Nausea/Vomiting

Syndrome Pathway(s)	Causes	Clinical Features	Antiemetic Management	Adjuvant
S Gastric stasis and gastric outflow obstruction **P** Vomiting center, gastrointestinal tract	Anticholinergic drugs, autonomic failure, ascites, hepatomegaly, tumor infiltration, peptic ulcer, gastritis	Epigastric fullness and discomfort. Early satiety. Flatulence, hiccough, acid reflux, and gastric regurgitation. Large volume emesis which may contain undigested food. Nausea often relieved by vomiting	Prokinetic Metoclopramide 10–20 mg TID PO 40–80 mg SQ infusion/24 hours	• Dietary advice • Paracentesis for ascites • Simethicone for flatulence • Steroid therapy may be used to improve the dysfunction induced by tumor infiltration of nerve plexuses • For total obstruction a venting gastrostomy or surgical bypass may be considered • H_2 blocker or proton pump inhibitor • Review drug regimen
S Stretch/irritation of visceral and gastrointestinal serosa **P** Vomiting center, gastrointestinal tract	Liver metastases, ureteric obstruction, tumor, constipation, bowel obstruction, lymph nodes	Pain is often a feature. Colic. Altered bowel habits. Nausea. Vomiting of fecal fluid in obstruction	Antihistamine DiphenhydrAMINE 25–50 mg TID or QID PO/IM/IV Promethazine 12.5–25 mg TID or QID PO/IM/IV/PR Hydroxyzine 25–100 mg TID or QID PO/IM	• Relieve the cause (e.g., constipation) with stimulant laxatives and enemas as required • Steroid therapy for the reduction of peri-tumor edema
S Raised intracranial pressure/meningism **P** Vomiting center	Cerebral tumor, intracranial tumor, intracranial bleeding, infiltration of meninges by tumor, skull metastases, cerebral infection	Neurological signs (e.g., drowsiness, dizziness, headache, nausea and/or vomiting, vomiting may be projectile in nature)	Antihistamine DiphenhydrAMINE 25–50 mg TID or QID PO/IM/IV Promethazine 12.5–25 mg TID or QID PO/IM/IV/PR Hydroxyzine 25–100 mg TID or QID PO/IM Anticholinergic Scopolamine Transdermal patch q 3 days	• High dose steroids may reduce cerebral edema and/or tumor mass • Bisphosphonates if hypercalcemia present

Editor's Note: **S** = Syndrome, **P** = Pathway(s)

(continued)

Table 3: Management of Nausea/Vomiting (continued)

Syndrome Pathway(s)	Causes	Clinical Features	Antiemetic Management	Adjuvant
S Pharyngeal stimulation **P** Vomiting center	Tenacious sputum not easily expectorated, infection (*Candida*)	Retching	Antihistamine DiphenhydrAMINE 25–50 mg TID or QID PO/IM/IV Promethazine 12.5–25 mg TID or QID PO/IM/IV/PR Hydroxyzine 25–100 mg TID or QID PO/IM	• Treat the cause. Saline nebulizers. Antibiotics • Antifungal therapy. If an inner ear problem, treat with meclizine
S Esophageal obstruction **P** Vomiting center	Tumor, odynophagia (painful swallowing), functional dysphagia, *Candida*	Regurgitation, dysphagia	Anticholinergic Will help to reduce saliva and secretions Scopolamine Transdermal patch q 3 days Octreotide	• Radiotherapy, brachiotherapy, laser therapy, high dose steroids, self-expanding stent, Celestin or Atkinson tube, surgery (not for patients with metastatic spread)
S Anxiety **P** Vomiting center	Psychological and emotional distress, anticipatory emesis associated with chemotherapy	Nausea, waves of nausea and vomiting, distraction may relieve symptoms	Antihistamine or Anticholinergics if required	• Address the anxiety with psychological techniques • Relaxation. Benzodiazepines. Ensure adequate pain control

1. Adapted with permission from: Campbell T, Hately J. The management of nausea and vomiting in advanced cancer. *International Journal of Palliative Nursing*. 2000;6(1):18–20, 22–25.
2. Editor's Note: **S** = Syndrome, **P** = Pathway(s)

XXII. Paresthesia and Neuropathy

A. **Definitions**

1. Paresthesia: a sensation of numbness, prickling or tingling; heightened sensitivity

2. Neuropathy: any disease of the nerves; may include sensory loss, muscle weakness and atrophy and decreased deep tendon reflexes

B. **Possible Etiologies**

1. Central and peripheral nerve lesions

2. Direct damage to peripheral and autonomic nerves

3. Metabolic and vascular changes of diabetes mellitus

4. Chemical or drug-induced: e.g., chemotherapy, isoniazid, alcohol

5. Amputation, AIDS, vitamin B-12 deficiency

6. Tumor invasion with pressure on nerves or plexuses

7. Spinal cord compression (considered an oncologic emergency)

C. **Assess for**

1. Sudden loss of sensation, motor function of lower extremities with or without loss of bladder or bowel control; **MAY INDICATE SPINAL CORD COMPRESSION WHICH IS A MEDICAL EMERGENCY.** Most common signs of pending cord compression are escalating back pain with or without bladder changes and before lower extremity weakness, worse when lying down, improved when standing. Amount of neurological deficit patient presents with is usually amount left with following treatment, therefore early recognition is imperative

2. Location and degree of numbness: patient's subjective descriptions of pain or sensation assist in determining etiology

3. Patient's course in the diseases process/trajectory for assistance in intervention planning

4. Patient safety in ambulation, ADLs

5. Patient and family understanding of cause of sudden change in sensation or motor function, need for safety in ambulation/ADLs, understanding of treatment options

D. **Potential Diagnoses**

1. Alteration in comfort related to peripheral sensory and neuropathic changes

2. Safety risk related to alteration in sensation

3. Patient and family knowledge deficit related to safety needs, medication effects, treatment options

4. Compromised patient and family coping related to uncontrolled pain

E. **Planning and Intervention: determining patient's course in disease process, trajectory will facilitate planning in the event of spinal cord compression**

1. If patient is in advanced stage of disease (weak, bed bound, poor nutritional status), symptom management may be appropriate option (i.e., steroids to decrease edema around cord; neuroleptic analgesia, opioids)

2. If patient is ambulatory, active and able to participate in self-care, palliative radiotherapy and steroids may provide significant benefit for quality of life

3. Tricyclic antidepressants (TCAs) are appropriate adjuvant analgesics to opioids for neuropathic pain (see Chapter IV, Section III. A. 1. d)

    a) Titrate dose every few days based upon the patient's response

    b) Therapeutic levels achieved in 3–7 days

4. Anticonvulsants can be considered for neuropathic pain

    a) If gabapentin: start low (e.g., 200–300 mg qHS). Dose can be titrated to 3600 mg daily maximum (in divided doses) for therapeutic effect

    b) If carbamazepine or phenytoin: monitor for effect and for drug interaction (monitor serum levels, CBC)

5. Appropriate bowel regimen if patient has decreased activity, is bed bound or has lost sensation in rectum

6. Foley catheter for urinary retention

7. Condom or Foley catheter for urinary incontinence if this causes skin irritation, patient anxiety and if patient/caregiver agree

8. Increase assistance with ADLs in home as indicated for patient personal needs and safety

F. Patient and Family Education

1. Expected medication effects and possible side effects

    a) Continue TCAs regularly

    (1) It takes 3–7 days to become therapeutic for neuropathic pain

    (2) Give at night, which might aid in sleeping and reduce daytime sedation

    b) Prepare patient and family to expect that gabapentin may cause sedation when initiated or dose increased

    c) Carbamazepine may cause dizziness, drowsiness, anorexia and nausea

    d) Phenytoin may cause ataxia, diplopia, dizziness, drowsiness

2. Safety needs when ambulating related to decreased sensation, motor ability and medication effects

G. Evaluate for effectiveness of interventions, specifically

1. Compliance with medication regimen

2. Effectiveness of medication and any side effects

3. Return of sensation, function

4. Safety needs/issues

H. Revise plan according to findings from ongoing evaluations, changes in patient status, or family needs

XXIII. Seizures

A. Definitions: usually intermittent tonic, clonic movements; convulsions caused by a large number of neurons discharging abnormally[17]

1. Primary (generalized) involving large parts of the brain and including grand mal and petit mal types

2. Focal (partial) involving specific regions of the brain with symptoms reflecting the location of the disturbance

B. **Possible Etiologies**[17]

1. Brain infarct, primary brain tumor or brain metastases, cerebral abscess, brain infection in HIV and AIDS

2. Increased intracranial pressure (may be associated with SIADH in some cancer patients)

3. Pre-existing seizure disorder

4. Medications (metabolites from normeperidine and propoxyphene) and their preservatives (sodium bisulfite); medications that lower seizure threshold include phenothiazines, butyrophenones, tricyclic antidepressants

5. Infection, stroke, hemorrhage, oxygen deprivation, paraneoplastic syndromes

6. Metabolic instability (hyponatremia, hypercalcemia, hypomagnesemia, hypoxemia, hypoglycemia)

7. Drug toxicity, drug withdrawal

C. **Assess for**

1. Acutely seizing patient: intervene with first intervention below

2. Underlying etiology reviewing medical history, disease process, current medications, history of trauma or recent fall, differentiate from myoclonus

3. Question patient and/or family to determine onset and type of seizure, presence of aura, headache, nausea and projectile vomiting

4. Drug levels if previously taking anticonvulsants; EEG may be warranted

5. Patient and family coping with seizure activity, their understanding of patient protection/ safety during seizure, medication effects and side effects

D. **Potential Diagnoses**

1. Safety precautions (e.g., risk for falls) for seizures from: etiology

2. Potential risk for medication toxicity or withdrawal side effects

    a) Dexamethasone is commonly given to those with seizure disorder; interaction between this drug and phenytoin is problematic, monitor phenytoin levels as appropriate

    b) Steroids must not be suddenly stopped: seizures may occur

3. Metabolic impairment related to hyponatremia, hypercalcemia, hypomagnesemia, hypoxia, hypoglycemia

4. Patient and family knowledge deficit related to etiology, disease process, medication effects/side effects, safety

E. **Planning and Intervention**

1. For actively seizing patient

    a) Assess airway, breathing, circulation and ensure adequate airway

    b) Protect patient from harm and ensure safety

c) Model calm demeanor

d) Medical therapy may include

(1) IV lorazepam (drug of choice)

(2) Diazepam enema, IV diazepam

(3) Fosphenytoin (Cerebyx®) IV

(4) Initiation of phenytoin, carbamazepine, valproic acid or phenobarbital[17]

2. Determine potentially treatable etiologies

a) Hypoglycemia: glucose PO/IV or glucagon SQ as indicated

b) Hyponatremia: fluid restriction, IV NaCl, adjustment of diuretics

c) Hypercalcemia: increase fluids PO/IV, pamidronate may be appropriate depending on disease trajectory

d) Hypoxemia: supplemental O_2; further evaluation of this etiology

e) Hypomagnesemia: supplemental magnesium

f) Infectious process (cerebral abscess, encephalitis, meningitis): antibiotics as indicated and according to patient's place on disease trajectory and advance directives

g) Substance abuse: support withdrawal, consult substance withdrawal specialist

F. **Patient and Family Education**

1. Anticipate potential for seizure activity and prepare family for patient safety, preemptive interventions, whom to call

2. Calmly rehearse, review caregiver interventions

3. Expected medication effects and potential side effects

G. **Evaluate**

1. Effectiveness of seizure management interventions

2. Family preparedness and coping

3. Patient safety

4. Medication effects and side effects

5. Blood draws to monitor levels of medications such as phenytoin

a) Phenytoin has a narrow therapeutic range, and drug interactions may lead to alterations in its plasma concentration

H. **Revise plan according to findings from ongoing evaluations, changes in patient status, or family needs**

XXIV. Urinary Incontinence/Retention[18]

A. **Definition: the inability to control urination**

B. **Possible Etiologies**

1. Urge incontinence: urge to void sensed, but cannot control urine flow long enough to reach toilet

    a) Due to bladder irritation such as infection, tumor, radiation, or chemotherapy

    b) Nervous system damage: spinal cord lesions (neurogenic bladder), stroke, multiple sclerosis, Parkinson's disease, Alzheimer's disease

    c) Decreased mobility or difficulty reaching the toilet in time

2. Stress incontinence: leakage of urine when intra-abdominal pressure is raised

    a) Damage or dysfunction of bladder sphincter due to

    (1) Tumor infiltration in genitourinary system or CNS or spinal cord lesions

    (2) Multiparity or post-menopausal changes in women

3. Overflow incontinence: bladder unable to empty normally

    a) Bladder outlet obstruction due to fecal mass, tumor, calculi, prostatic hypertrophy

    b) Detrusor muscle failure due to anticholinergic drugs, CNS lesions, or debility and confusion

4. Functional incontinence: an involuntary or unpredictable passage of urine with no impairment of the genitourinary tract

    a) Cognitive dysfunction: depression leading to self-neglect, confusion, excessive sedation

    b) Mobility or functional problems: immobility, unable to undress, inaccessible toilet facilities, final stage of illness

5. Many drugs can lead to any of the aforementioned urinary incontinence problems

    a) Diuretics increase volume and frequency

    b) Sedatives decrease awareness of need to void, as well as decrease bladder contraction and outlet resistance

    c) Anticholinergics decrease bladder contraction

    d) Antiparkinsonian drugs increase outlet resistance

6. Metabolic disorders: hypercalcemia

7. Atonic bladder: no awareness of bladder fullness or urgency

    a) Diabetic neuropathy

    b) Spinal cord lesions or cord compression

    c) Neurologic dysfunction

8. Fistula

C. **Assess for**

1. History, including nature and duration of symptoms, medications, recent treatments for cancer

2. Physical exam: bladder distention, perineal swelling, fecal impaction, simple neurologic exam (including sensation and sensorimotor deficits), signs of hypercalcemia, functional assessment (mobility, able to dress/undress self, presence of aphasia or dysphasia), skin assessment

3. Urge incontinence: nocturia, frequency with urination

4. Stress incontinence: leakage of urine upon laughing, coughing, sneezing, lifting or bending

5. Overflow incontinence: bladder distention, discomfort, urgency, continual dribbling and only voiding small amounts, large residual urine after voiding, fecal impaction

6. Functional incontinence: mobility, ability to perform ADLs, cognitive level, depression

D. **Diagnoses**

1. Altered urinary elimination related to anatomic dysfunction or obstruction, medications, or metabolic disorder

2. Urinary incontinence, urge, related to bladder irritation, sensory-motor disorder, or decreased mobility

3. Urinary incontinence, stress, related to decrease in bladder or sphincter support

4. Urinary incontinence, functional, related to cognitive dysfunction or mobility problems

5. Risk for impaired skin integrity related to urinary incontinence

6. Patient and family knowledge deficit related to etiology and management of urinary incontinence

7. Patient and family anxiety related to urinary incontinence

8. Risk for falls trying to get to the bathroom

E. **Planning and Intervention**

1. Review medications and discontinue those that may be causing incontinence (if appropriate). Medications that can cause urinary incontinence include opioids, sedatives, antidepressants, antipsychotics, antiparkinsonian drugs and alpha-adrenergic blocking agents[18]

2. If appropriate, establish a regular voiding schedule (i.e., every 2 hours)

3. Alter environment to make toileting easier (i.e., move patient closer to toilet, or utilize a bedside commode, urinal, or bedpan, assuring modesty and dignity is maintained)

4. Decrease fluid intake at night, and limit intake of food/fluids containing caffeine or alcohol

5. If fecal impaction is present, disimpact and teach bowel regime to patient and family to avoid further problems

6. Consider catheterizing, either indwelling or external

7. Utilize incontinence supplies, such as pads, briefs, etc.

8. Teach patient and family hygiene and skin care measures

9. Urge incontinence: oxybutynin (Ditropan®) or tolterodine (Detrol®) (long acting products preferred). Antibiotics for UTI, urinary tract analgesics such as phenazopyridine (Pyridium®) for pain, imipramine for neurogenic bladder[18]

10. Stress incontinence: teach pelvic floor muscle exercises (PFME) and voiding schedule, pessary, imipramine at bedtime for anticholinergic effect

11. Overflow incontinence: discontinue anticholinergic medications, if possible; disimpact if necessary; cholinergic drug such as bethanechol (Urecholine®); indwelling catheterization if obstruction persists

12. Functional incontinence: interventions rely on cause of incontinence; indwelling catheter may be only choice

13. Incontinence related to fistulas is treated by establishing voiding schedules, catheterization, and, if indicated, urinary diversion (if life expectancy is not short)

F. Patient and Family Education

1. Expected medication effects and potential side effects

2. Demonstrate correct hygiene and skin care techniques to prevent skin breakdown

3. Explain correct catheter care and signs of catheter malfunction

4. Explain safety measures if altering environment for ease in toileting (i.e., have patient call for assistance, voiding schedules, assuring clear path to bathroom)

5. Explain signs and symptoms of urinary tract infection (UTI)

G. Evaluate

1. Effectiveness of interventions (Are patient and family satisfied with outcome?)

2. Skin integrity

3. Medication effects and side effects

4. Patient safety

H. Revise plan according to findings from ongoing evaluations, changes in patient and family needs

CITED REFERENCES

1. Bergstrom N, Bennett MA, Carlson CE, et al. *Pressure Ulcer Treatment: Clinical Practice Guideline. Quick Reference Guide for Clinicians, No. 15*. Rockville, MD: U.S. Department of Health and Human Services, Public Health Service, Agency for Health Care Policy and Research; 1994.

2. Dahlin CM, Goldsmith T. Dysphagia, xerostomia, and hiccups. In: Ferrell BR, Coyle N, eds. *Textbook of Palliative Nursing*. 2nd ed. New York, NY: Oxford University Press; 2006:195–218.

3. Waller A, Caroline NL. *Handbook of Palliative Care in Cancer*. 2nd ed. Boston, MA: Butterworth-Heinemann; 2000.

4. Rhiner M, Slatkin NE. Pruritus, fever, and sweats, In: Ferrell BR, Coyle N, eds. *Textbook of Palliative Nursing*. 2nd ed. New York, NY: Oxford University Press; 2006:345–363.

5. Kuebler KK, Heidrich DE, Vena C, English N. Delirium, confusion, and agitation. In: Ferrell BR, Coyle N, eds. *Textbook of Palliative Nursing*. New York, NY: Oxford University Press; 2006:401–420.

6. Collins CA. Ascites. *Clinical Journal of Oncology Nursing*. 2001;5(1):43–44.

7. Kemp C. *Terminal Illness: A Guide to Nursing Care*. 2nd ed. Philadelphia, PA: Lippincott; 1999.

8. Letizia M, Norton E. Successful management of malignant bowel obstruction. *Journal of Hospice and Palliative Nursing*. 2002;5(3):152–158.

9. Larson PD, Mallett L. Gastrointestinal symptoms. In: Matzo ML, Sherman DW, eds. *Palliative Care Nursing: Quality Care to the End of Life*. New York, NY: Springer Publishing Company; 2010: 463–487.

10. Dudgeon D. Dyspnea, death rattle, and cough. In: Ferrell BR, Coyle N, eds. *Textbook of Palliative Nursing*. New York, NY: Oxford University Press; 2006:319–344.

11. Runyan BA. *AASLD Practice Guidelines: Management of Adult Patients with Ascites Due to Cirrhosis: An Update*. 2009. Available at: aasld.org/practiceguidelines/Documents/Bookmarked%20Practice%20Guidelines/Ascites%20Update6-2009.pdf. Accessed February 3, 2010.

12. Anderson PR, Dean GE. Fatigue. In: Ferrell BR, Coyle N, eds. *Textbook of Palliative Nursing*. New York, NY: Oxford University Press; 2006:155–168.

13. Chochinov HM, Breitbart W. *Handbook of Psychiatry in Palliative Care*. 2nd ed. New York, NY: Oxford University Press; 2009.

14. McCaffery M, Pasero C. *Pain: Clinical Manual*. St. Louis, MO: Mosby; 1999.

15. Miller K, Miller M. Managing common gastrointestinal symptoms at the end of life. *Journal of Hospice and Palliative Nursing*. 2002;4(1):34–42.

16. Campbell T, Hately J. The management of nausea and vomiting in advanced cancer. *International Journal of Palliative Nursing*. 2000;6(1):18–20, 22–25.

17. Paice JA. Neurological disturbances. In: Ferrell BR, Coyle N, eds. *Textbook of Palliative Nursing*. 2nd ed. New York, NY: Oxford University Press; 2006:365–373.

18. Gray M, Campbell F. Urinary tract disorders. In: Ferrell BR, Coyle N, eds. *Textbook of Palliative Nursing*. 2nd ed. New York, NY: Oxford University Press; 2006:265–283.

ADDITIONAL REFERENCES AND RESOURCES

Brajtman S. Helping the family through the experience of terminal restlessness. *Journal of Hospice and Palliative Nursing.* 2005;7(2):73–81.

Corless IB, Nicholas PK, Davis SM, Dolan SA, McGibbon CA. Symptom status, medication adherence, and quality of life in HIV disease. *Journal of Hospice and Palliative Nursing.* 2005;7(3):129–138.

FAST FACTS and Concepts. End of Life/Palliative Education Resource Center (EPERC). Available at: www.eperc.mcw.edu/. Accessed December 17, 2009.

Ferrell BR, Coyle N, eds. *Textbook of Palliative Nursing.* 2nd ed. New York, NY: Oxford University Press; 2010.

Ferris F, von Gunten C. Fast Facts #40: Pressure ulcer management: prevention (part 1), 2nd ed. End of Life Palliative Education Resource Center (EPERC). Available at: www.eperc.mcw.edu/. Accessed December 18, 2009.

Houseman G. Symptom management of the patient with amyotrophic lateral sclerosis: a guide for hospice nurses. *Journal of Hospice and Palliative Nursing.* 2008;10(4):207–213.

Jablonski A. Level of symptom relief and the need for palliative care in the hemodialysis population. *Journal of Hospice and Palliative Nursing.* 2007;9(1):50–58.

Jablonski A, Wyatt GK. A model for identifying barriers to effective symptom management at the end of life. *Journal of Hospice and Palliative Nursing.* 2005;7(1):23–36.

Kazanowski M. Family caregivers' medication management of symptoms in patients with cancer near death. *Journal of Hospice and Palliative Nursing.* 2005;7(3):174–181.

Lentz J, McMillan SC. The impact of opioid-induced constipation on patients near the end of life: perspectives of patients, family caregivers, and nurses. *Journal of Hospice and Palliative Nursing.* 2010;12(1):29–38.

Little L, Dionne B, Eaton J. Nursing assessment of depression among palliative care cancer patients. *Journal of Hospice and Palliative Nursing.* 2005;7(2):98–106.

McMillan SC, Dunbar SB, Zhang W. The prevalence of symptoms in hospice patients with end-stage heart disease. *Journal of Hospice and Palliative Nursing.* 2007;9(3):124–131.

McMillan SC, Dunbar SB, Zhang W. Validation of the hospice quality-of-life index and the constipation assessment scale in end-stage cardiac disease patients in hospice care. *Journal of Hospice and Palliative Nursing.* 2008;10(2):106–117.

Quijada E, Billings JA. Fast Facts #60: Pharmacologic management of delirium: update on newer agents. End-of-Life Physician Education Resource Center. Available at: www.eperc.mcw.edu/. Accessed December 18, 2009.

Smitz LL, Woods AB. Prevalence, severity, and correlates of depressive symptoms on admission to inpatient hospice. *Journal of Hospice and Palliative Nursing.* 2006;8(2):86–91.

Treece P. Standardized Order Sets for End of Life Care. *Journal of Hospice and Palliative Nursing.* 2007;9(2):70–71.

von Gunten C, Ferris F. Fast Facts #37: Pruritus. End-of-Life Physician Education Resource Center. Available at: www.eperc.mcw.edu/. Accessed December 18, 2009.

Weissman DE. Fast Facts #27: Dyspnea at end of life. End-of-Life Physician Education Resource Center. Available at: www.eperc.mcw.edu/. Accessed December 18, 2009.

Wrede-Seaman L. *Symptom Management Algorithms: A Handbook for Palliative Care.* 3rd ed. Yakima, WA: Intellicard; 2009.

CHAPTER VI

COMMUNICATING AT THE END OF LIFE

Beth Miller Kraybill BSN, CHPN® MDiv.
Mary Ersek, PhD, RN, FAAN, FPCN
Marty Richards, MSW, LICSW

Adapted from: Ersek M, Richards M. Communicating at the end of life. In: Ersek M, ed. *Core Curriculum for the Hospice and Palliative Nursing Assistant*. Dubuque, IA: Kendall Hunt Publishing; 2003:59–69.

I. **Basic Concepts of Communication**

   A. **Defining Communication**

      1. Communication: exchange of information in which meaning is shared

      2. Communication has two parts: sending and receiving

      3. Communication is both verbal and nonverbal

   B. **Verbal Communication**

      1. What someone says

      2. Also includes other verbalizations, for example, moans, groans, sighs

      3. When people have lost their ability to speak because of aphasia or other problems, their ability to understand and respond in ways other than verbal often remains good; do not assume a lack of understanding

   C. **Nonverbal Communication**

      1. Nonverbal communication includes

         a) Posture and positioning (sitting, standing, reclining)

         b) Gestures

         c) Body movements

         d) Facial expressions

         e) Tone of voice

         f) Appearance (e.g., clothing, hair, jewelry, etc.)

g) Eye contact (or lack of eye contact)

h) Touch (or lack of touch)

2. Touch

   a) Important nonverbal communication skill

   b) For some people, gentle touch communicates support, respect, care

   c) For others, touch invades personal space and is threatening

   d) Let the other person take the lead; watch the person's response to initial touch to decide whether to use this communication approach

3. The role of silence in communication[1]

   a) Silence does not necessarily mean the person is reluctant to talk; may mean that they are in deep thought about something painful or sensitive; sit quietly and attentively; give the person time to respond

   b) Sometimes you may not know what to say; at other times, there are no adequate words; in these situations, saying nothing and remaining close can offer comfort; this is called *presence* or *being present*

   c) Learn to be comfortable with silence; a non-anxious presence is especially important when working with patients and families at the end of life

D. Basic Communication Skills: Setting the Environment

1. Ensure that the person can see you, especially your face

2. If possible, get at eye level with the person

3. Go to or create a quiet, private place; ask to turn off the radio or TV; close door if appropriate

4. Take into account vision and hearing problems that may hinder communication

E. Basic Communication Skills: Listening[2-3]

1. An active process of receiving, paying attention to, and making meaning of what another person is communicating

2. To listen, you must stop talking

3. Guide for listening

   a) Face the person and maintain eye contact, if culturally appropriate

   b) Make sure your nonverbal communication "says" to the person "I am listening" (i.e., lean toward the person, nod your head, murmur "mmm," keep your arms open, relaxed and not crossed)

   c) Acknowledge what the person is telling you by making comments such as, "I see," or, "tell me more"

   d) Make sure you understand what you are hearing; ask the person to clarify if necessary, but try not to interrupt; restate what you heard (i.e., "You're feeling overwhelmed" or "You are angry at the doctor.")

F. **Basic Communication Skills: Speaking**

1. Introduce yourself routinely; be sure that the person you are speaking with understands who you are and your role

2. Speak clearly and unhurriedly

3. Use clear words and simple sentences; ask if the person has questions

4. Avoid distracting behaviors (e.g., pacing while you talk or listen, frowning, finger tapping, or checking your watch)

5. If necessary, repeat ideas and instructions

6. Use open ended questions

G. **Cultural Differences in Communication (also see Chapter VII)**

1. Different cultures may have different rules about communication; for example, culture influences whether to make eye contact

2. Culture influences communication style; for example, some cultures favor direct, to-the-point communication; other cultures favor indirect communication, that is, they may talk in general about being sick instead of directly stating that the person has cancer

3. Some cultures use more expressive communication styles, that is, active facial expressions and gestures; other cultures are less expressive

4. Words have multiple meanings

    a) Words that have one meaning for a particular group may have a different meaning in another culture; for example, for middle-class, European-Americans "illness" may refer to a state of poor health brought about by a disease or stress; to someone from a traditional culture, illness may be a state of poor health caused by a curse or a behavior

    b) Some words have no direct translation of some words into English or another language

    c) Do not make assumptions; ask the person what he or she means by certain words, such as "illness," "family," "faith," or "care"

5. There may also be different expectations about with whom to communicate (e.g., the eldest son may be the designated decision-maker in the family)

6. Culture also influences how directly death is discussed

    a) Some cultures believe that talking about death will hasten its occurrence

    b) Cultural norms can clash when people are asked to make end-of-life decisions, such as hospice or palliative care; cultural differences also impact discussion of advance directives (i.e., living wills); if such obstacles arise, be sure to utilize all team members for support

7. Cultural guides (i.e., books, websites, resource persons) can provide information on general priorities and expectations within communities; however

    a) There is no "cookbook" about how to talk to everyone in a culture

    b) Find out all you can about a cultural group, but remember that each person is an individual and each family is unique

c) Ask the patient or family what their traditions are. Many families appreciate the opportunity to share and teach

8. Work with a medical interpreter if English is not the family's or patient's first language; avoid using family members as translators

H. Gender Differences in Communication

1. Men and women have different styles in how they share information and feelings
2. Culture and religion also affect social status of men and women, which in turn influences how they expect others to communicate with them
3. Older women in particular may defer to a husband or son in making decisions or talking about concern

I. Age

1. All communication with children must take into account their stage of development; for instance do they understand abstract words like "terminal?" If they understand the word, do they have the emotional maturity to deal with its meaning?
2. In many cultures, older adults are treated with great respect; communication must reflect this respect
3. Ask the older adult how she or he prefers to be addressed, for example, do they like to be called "Mrs. Hernandez" or "Maria"?
4. Advanced age increases the chance that sensory losses (e.g., hearing or eyesight) will influence communication

J. Awareness of One's Own Communication Style

1. Know your own personal communication style so you can understand where your style may create difficulties for others; if conflicts arise, seek assistance from the team
2. Avoid labeling others when their communication style differs from yours (e.g., labeling a quiet person as withdrawn; labeling an assertive person as pushy or threatening)

II. Elements of Therapeutic Communication: Special Issues in Working with the Dying

A. Effective communication is an essential skill for working with those at the end of life

B. Challenges in Communicating with Dying Patients[2]

1. Cultural and societal issues

   a) Denial of death; although our society is becoming more open, there still is a reluctance to speak openly about death, particularly to the dying person

   b) Little or no experience with death; many Americans have never witnessed a death or spent time with a dying person and have a knowledge deficit

2. Patients' and families' fears and emotions (see following section)

3. Concerns of the care provider

   a) Fears of

      (1) Not knowing what to say

      (2) Fear of not knowing "the answer"

      (3) Making a mistake and upsetting the patient and family

      (4) Discomfort with conflict or other peoples strong emotions

      (5) Personal fear of dying

4. Conditions that make communication difficult, such as stroke, dementia, hearing and vision problems or sleepiness and confusion resulting from disease and medications

C. **Common Patient and Family Fears and Emotions at the End of Life That Affect Communication**[4]

   1. Fear

      a) Of having pain and other distressing symptoms

      b) Of dying alone

      c) That caregivers will not give good care

      d) Of losing one's mind, losing control

      e) About the dying process, death, afterlife

      f) About losing relationships

      g) About losing one's identity (i.e., mother, daughter, employee, etc.)

      h) About money, loss of income

      i) About being a burden (physically, emotionally, and financially)

   2. Anger

      a) At the effects (physical, emotional, and social) of the illness

      b) At others in the family and network of friends

      c) At the financial losses

      d) At the loss of plans and dreams

      e) At the fact that their loved one is leaving them

      f) That the person at the end of life chooses to confide in someone other than them

   3. Guilt

      a) At what they should have done

      b) At what they did in the past

      c) For needing time away from their loved one or for not being with their loved one more

      d) At losing their temper

e) For unresolved relationships

f) About turning over the care of their loved one to a non-family member (respite care, hospitalization, nursing home placement, etc.)

4. Sadness

a) Underlies everything and can be overwhelming

b) Occurs often and can get worse with each new loss

5. Confusion: facing so many changes and feeling they are unable to keep up; difficulty accepting that the patient's condition is changing and the prognosis is uncertain

6. Hopelessness and helplessness: feeling that there is nothing that can be done about a situation; lack of control over a situation; anger can be the outward response to feelings of helplessness and hopelessness

7. Inability to accept that loved one is dying; sometimes family members refuse to discuss dying or hospice care with the dying patient

8. Laughter, love, and joy

a) These can still be shared

b) Humor is a gift to one's sanity

c) Often sharing something "spiritual" is a way to connect

D. Therapeutic Communication with Dying Patients and Their Families: Basic Concepts

1. Being present is more important than "saying the right thing:" often there is nothing to say

2. Encourage patients and families to reminisce and tell their stories[1]

a) Provides reassurance that their lives have meaning

b) Helps to take the focus off the present difficulties that patients and families are facing

c) Be ready and willing to listen to the sadness that may come with reminiscing

3. Care providers do not have all the answers; it's okay to say "I do not know."

4. Important messages to communicate: (adapted from Module 6: Communication, ELNEC project; 2009)

a) "I will listen to you."

b) "I will be honest and truthful with you."

c) "I will not abandon you."

d) "I value you as a person."

e) "I will respect your values and goals and help you to achieve those goals as much as I am able."

f) "I will give you every chance to ask questions. If I do not know the answer to your question, I'll try to find someone who does have the answer."

g) "I accept that you will at times be sad, frightened, or angry. I will not turn away or avoid you when you are experiencing these emotions."

h) "When caring for you or your loved one, I will ask myself, 'What would I do if this were my family member?'"

5. Other helpful messages for caregivers and family to communicate to people before they die[4]

   a) "I love you"

   b) "Thank you"

   c) "I forgive you"

   d) "Please forgive me"

   e) "Goodbye"

6. Maintain a good match between verbal and nonverbal messages; for example, telling the patient that they can trust you, but often failing to answer their call light is <u>not</u> a good match between words and actions

E. **Timing**

   1. Make sure that someone is physically comfortable before you begin a conversation

   2. Be aware of the times that patients want to talk about certain things; respect their wishes when they do not want to talk; use their timetables, not your own

   3. Watch medication times for the most pain-free opportunities to talk

   4. Anticipate teachable moments when families and patients are most open to talking

F. **Asking Questions**

   1. Remember that people have limited energy for things that have little importance to them

   2. Limit questions by focusing on the patient's or family's concerns; do not ask questions if you really do not need or want to know the answer

   3. Questions should show that you are really interested in the patient's situation

   4. Remember to respect the privacy of the person's feelings, one of the few things they have left

   5. If you need to ask a sensitive question, explain why you are asking the question

G. **Fostering hope without making false assurances**[5]

   1. Many providers wonder how they can help patients and families maintain hope at the end of life

   2. The end of life can seem like a hopeless time because the hope for a cure is destroyed; however, research shows that hope often is maintained and can increase at the end of life[6–8]

   3. How providers interact with patients and families can increase or decrease their hope

   4. Hope can be thought of as having four dimensions[9]

      a) Experiential: dimension in which people accept and move beyond their current suffering to find joy and meaning

      b) Rational thought: thinking, planning process in which people make goals and take steps to meet those goals; goals can be short-term (e.g., to have pain managed during family visits) or long term (e.g., to live until a grandson's graduation); goals change as disease progresses

c) Relational: connectedness with others; people can become more or less hopeful, depending on their relationships; for example, being cut off from close family members can decrease hope

d) Spiritual: Involves people looking outside of themselves at the greater whole, something "bigger" than themselves; spirituality may involve religious beliefs focused on a deity, and also includes people's connection to nature or the universe

5. Ways to support patients' and families' hope at the end of life[3,5]

a) Experiential: prevent and treat end-of-life symptoms; use humor as appropriate; support patient and family in using positive self-talk (e.g., "We are strong," "We can handle this," "We are together in this"); encourage reminiscing; help engagement in meaningful aesthetic activities such as playing or listening to music or doing art

b) Rational thinking: assist patient and family to identify, obtain and revise specific goals; help in identifying resources to meet goals; help patient and family maintain a sense of control; provide accurate information about the patient's condition; help patient and family identify past successes

c) Relational: provide time for patient's relationships; affirm patient and family's self-worth; establish and maintain an open, respectful connection; assure the patient and family that you accept them and will not abandon them

d) Spiritual: help patient and family participate in religious rituals; facilitate visits with clergy; willingly participate in conversation related to the meaning of life and death and other existential questions

H. Patients' communication at the end of life[10]

1. Often, dying patients and their families need to share memories and emotions

2. Sometimes people use symbols to express their feelings or their understandings about their own living and dying; this is often referred to as near death awareness; for example

   a) Talk about meeting and talking with others who have died before them

   b) Insist that the dead person is "waiting for me"

   c) Talk about needing to get "a ticket for the train"

   d) Indicates that death is near and that he or she is ready to die

3. Some patients may need to talk with others to settle relationships and apologize for past actions

I. Educating and Supporting Families and Patients in Terminal Illness

1. Help people understand the importance of open communication at the end of life

2. Education can take place formally and informally

3. Educate and support patients and families by role modeling effective communication skills

4. Use written materials so the patient and family have a resource to review

5. Provide information in ways that empower the family; acknowledge resistance and affirm readiness—these are both necessary coping mechanisms

III. Dealing with Conflict[3]

   A. **The crisis of a terminal illness can bring issues to the surface and result in open family conflicts; you may get caught right in the middle of it; remember that in these situations**

   1. There are many sides to every situation
   2. Do not take sides
   3. Remember that you see only a snapshot in the whole moving picture of the family's interactions
   4. Sometimes, conflict is expressed to or directed at other family members because these people are "safe" and patients know that they will be forgiven as part of unconditional love that exists in the families
   5. Grief can be expressed as anger
   6. Sometimes, anger is directed at healthcare team members

   B. **Dealing with patient or family anger directed at healthcare provider**

   1. Tips for managing your own responses[3]

      a) Take an emotional step back from the situation; if you can, physically get away from the situation
      b) Think about your emotions: what exactly are you feeling? Anger? Fear? Sadness? Something else?
      c) Do any of the emotions you are feeling show themselves in your actions? How?
      d) Talk with other team members about how you are feeling; together, try to figure out what the conflict is about and who is involved
      e) Talk with the other people involved in the conflict; make a plan for dealing with the conflict or disagreement
      f) Use "I" statements (e.g., "I am trying to understand what you would like me to do," or "I feel uncomfortable when you raise your voice")

   2. When you communicate with someone who is angry or distressed, remember the following[2]

      a) Treat the person with respect
      b) Recognize frustrating and frightening situations; put yourself in the person's situation. How would you feel? How would you want to be treated?
      c) Answer the person's questions clearly; if you cannot answer the questions say so; then consult with other team members and get back to the person
      d) Keep the person informed; tell the person what you are going to do and why
      e) Do not keep the person waiting for long periods; address the person's questions and concerns as quickly as possible
      f) Stay calm; our non-anxious, attentive presence is more powerful than your words
      g) Recognize that families and patients need to express their grief and frustration; remember that anger is a normal part of the grieving process

h) Do not argue with or touch the person within the midst of the conflict

i) Use active listening skills; let the person express angry feelings; it is acceptable to set limits on abuse behavior

j) Protect yourself from violent behaviors by standing at a safe distance, or leaving the area if necessary

k) Report the person's behavior to other team members and enlist their support in problem-solving

CITED REFERENCES

1. American Association of Colleges of Nursing and the City of Hope National Medical Center. *Module 6: Communication. End-of-Life Nursing Education Consortium (ELNEC) Project*. 2009. Funded through the Robert Wood Johnson Foundation.

2. Sorrentino S, Gorek B. *Mosby's Textbook for Long-Term Care Assistants*, 4th ed. St. Louis, MO: Mosby; 2003:76, 88–95.

3. Richards M, Ersek M. *Communication at the End-of-Life. Palliative Care Resource Education Team (PERT) Train-The-Trainer Curriculum*. Seattle, WA: Swedish Medical Center; 2004.

4. Byock I. *Dying Well: The Prospects for Growth at the End of Life*. New York, NY: Riverhead Books; 1997.

5. Ersek M. The meaning of hope in the dying. In: Ferrell BR, Coyle N, eds. *Textbook of Palliative Nursing*. 2nd ed. New York, NY: Oxford University Press; 2006:513–529.

6. Herth K. Fostering hope in terminally-ill people. *J Adv Nurs*. 1990;15:1250–1259.

7. Herth K. Hope in the family caregiver of terminally-ill people. *J Adv Nurs*. 1993;18:538–548.

8. Ritchie MA. Self-esteem and hopefulness in adolescents with cancer. *J Pediatr Nurs*. 2001;16:35–42.

9. Farran CJ, Herth KA, Popovich JM. *Hope and Hopelessness: Critical Clinical Concepts*. Thousand Oaks, CA: Sage; 1995.

10. Callanan M, Kelley P. *Final Gifts: Understanding the Special Awareness, Needs, & Communications of the Dying*. New York, NY: Bantam Books; 1997.

ADDITIONAL REFERENCES AND RESOURCES

Dalinis PM. Informed consent and decisional capacity. *Journal of Hospice and Palliative Nursing*. 2005;(1):52–57.

Glass E, Cluxton D. Truth-telling: ethical issues in clinical practice. *Journal of Hospice and Palliative Nursing*. 2004;6(4):232–242.

Rosenblum D. Listening to people with cancer. *Sem Oncol*. 1994;12(21):701–704.

Schirm V, Sheehan DK. Conversations about choices for end-of-life care: knowing and understanding preferences. *Journal of Hospice and Palliative Nursing*. 2005;7(2):91–97.

Zen Hospice Project [website]. Available at: www.zenhospice.org.

CHAPTER VII

CULTURAL CONSIDERATIONS IN END-OF-LIFE CARE

Sarah A. Wilson, PhD, RN

I. **Culture**

   A. **Definitions**

   1. There are many different definitions of culture. Culture was first defined in 1871 by Edward Tylor, a British anthropologist, as the complex whole, which includes knowledge, beliefs, art, morals, law, custom, and any other capabilities, and habits acquired by a person as a member of society[1]

   2. Culture is the behaviors and beliefs that are learned and shared by members of a group[2]

   3. Culture is a way of perceiving, behaving, and evaluating the environment and provides a blueprint for determining values, beliefs, and practices[3]

   4. Culture is a blueprint for values, beliefs, and practices

   B. **Characteristics of Culture**[3-5]

   1. Culture functions as a whole, a change in one part affects the other parts

   2. Culture is socially learned and shared by members of a group; certain values and ideas are shared. Culture is not transmitted genetically

   3. Culture is dynamic and constantly changing. Culture enables humans to adapt to changes in the environment, resources, and technology

   4. Culture is universal; all humans have culture

   5. Culture often exists at an unconscious level or implicit level

   6. People may belong to more than one cultural group. Culture may include a religious group, a professional group, age group, or an ethnic group. For example, someone may be a member of the Roman Catholic culture, the culture of vocational nurse, a baby-boomer or a member of the Asian culture

   7. Cultures share common characteristics. One culture is not better than another culture

C. **Concepts and Terminology Related to Culture**[4-6]

1. Acculturation

    a) The process of adapting to another culture, modifying or changing one's culture as a result of contact with another culture. Example, changing language to speak English

    b) Factors that may influence acculturation are age, education, length of time in this country, income or socioeconomic status, and religion

2. Diversity

    a) Refers to difference in race, ethnicity, national origin, age, religion, gender, sexual orientation, social and economic class or status, education and related attributes of groups of people[5]

3. Ethnicity or ethnic group[4]

    a) Refers to groups whose members share a common social and cultural heritage that is passed down to each generation

    b) Members of an ethnic group have a sense of "shared people hood," or a sense of a common identity

    c) Answers question "Who am I?"

4. Ethnocentrism

    a) The tendency for people to believe their ways of thinking, acting, and believing are the only right and proper ways[5]

5. Prejudice

    a) Unjustified negative attitude based on a person's group membership

6. Race[4-6]

    a) Concept that refers to physical and biological differences. Members of a group that share certain physical traits such as skin color, bone structure, or blood

    b) Concept of biological race is not consistent with scientific data and does not explain human variation

    c) All humans are very similar, 99.9% at the DNA level

    d) Race has been used to classify people into groups and treat certain groups unfairly

7. Racism

    a) Belief that members of one race are superior to another race

    b) Has been described as prejudice combined with power

    c) May be overt or covert

    d) Implies that superior or inferior traits are determined by race

8. Stereotype

    a) Belief that all people from a given group are the same and share the same values and beliefs or characteristics

D. **Why Is Culture Important to Study?**[4,7,8]

1. Changing population demographics in the United States

    a) White majority population is aging and shrinking. The Black, Hispanic, Asian, and American Indian populations are young and growing[4]

    (1) White 80%

    (2) Black or African American 12.8%

    (3) American Indian and Alaska Native 1%

    (4) Asian 4.4%

    (5) Hispanic or Latino of any race 15.1%

    b) By 2030 more than 40% of the U.S. population will be members of diverse racial and ethnic groups[8]

    c) Immigration patterns into the United States have changed. Prior to the 1940s most immigrants were from Europe. New immigrants are from Mexico, Philippines, China, India, Brazil, Pakistan, Japan, Turkey, Egypt, and Thailand[4]

2. Cultural identity is integral to all aspects of life

3. Culture influences how people define health and illness, who they consult for health problems, how they care for the sick, and the practices used to stay healthy

4. Beliefs about death and dying are an integral part of culture

5. Helps us to plan and deliver care that is culturally sensitive and appropriate

6. Helps us to learn about our own culture and how it influences our behavior

II. **Cultural Sensitivity and Cultural Competence**[2,4,5,9,10]

A. **Cultural sensitivity and cultural competence are different**

1. Cultural sensitivity is an awareness of differences among groups. Relates to personal attitudes such as not saying things that are offensive

2. Cultural competence is the incorporation of one's cultural diversity experience, awareness, and sensitivity into everyday practice behaviors. It goes beyond cultural awareness or sensitivity. Culture competence combines knowledge, attitudes, acquired skills, and behavior. It is an approach

    a) Culturally competent healthcare providers

    (1) Are willing to learn and ask questions

    (2) Keep an open mind, avoid making assumptions and judgments

    (3) Learn from mistakes

    (4) Appreciate differences in people

    (5) Recognize building relationships takes time

    (6) Have a desire to be culturally competent

B. **Culturally competent healthcare is based on the uniqueness of a person's culture; includes cultural norms and values**

C. **Barriers to cultural competence**
1. Biases, known and unconscious
2. Lack of knowledge of other cultures
3. Lack of desire to become culturally competent
4. Lack of exposure to other cultures

III. **Cultural Values in the United States**

A. **Dominant Values**
1. Achievement and success
2. Competition
3. Freedom
4. Individualism and individuals making decisions
5. Work
6. Progress
7. Youth and beauty
8. Volunteerism, helping others in times of need

B. **Values of U.S. Healthcare System**
1. Scientific medicine, based on scientific facts
2. Use of technology to treat disease or stop progression of disease
3. Cure, the ability to eliminate or correct the problem
4. Autonomy and truth telling, informing the patient of the nature of the illness and the likelihood of recovery
5. Efficiency

IV. **Models for Cultural Assessment**[3-5]

A. **A cultural assessment may be defined as a systematic appraisal of individuals, groups, and communities**

B. **A number of different models exist for a cultural assessment**

C. **Most models include information about communication, nutrition, education, family patterns, religious preference, ethnic affiliation, time perceptions, space and biological variations**

D. **The four C's of culture**

1. C = Call: What do you call your problem? What do you think is wrong? Why did this happen to you?

2. C = Cause: What do you think caused the problem?

3. C = Cope: How do you cope with the problem?

4. C = Concerns: What concerns do you have about problem? The treatment? How serious do you think it is?

E. **Fong's[3] CONFHER model is practical and easy to use. CONFHER includes[3]**

1. C = Communication

    a) Does the patient read and speak English? Does the patient understand common health terms such as "pain" or "fever"?

    b) Is an interpreter needed?

    c) Nonverbal behavior such as facial expression, eye contact when speaking, body language, and comfortable space between individuals when talking

    d) Examples of communication: Native Americans avoid eye contact and value silence. Japanese Americans bow head when greeting to show respect and speak softly. African Americans are very expressive in communication

2. O = Orientation

    a) What is the person's ethnic identity, value orientation, and acculturation?

    b) What group does the person identify with? For example, Asian, Chinese, African American?

    c) Where were they born?

    d) What is their value orientation?

        (1) Relationship of humans and nature

        (2) Purpose in life

        (3) Time orientation. Past, present or future oriented?

    e) Examples of orientation. American Indians value the past and believe humans should live in harmony with nature

3. N = Nutrition

    a) Food preferences and taboos

    b) Meaning of food, association with certain events or celebrations. For example, people may have special food for Christmas, Chanukah, or birthdays

    c) Food is source of comfort and love

    d) Ask people if there are any foods that they must avoid. For example, eating pork is a taboo for Jewish or Muslim persons

4. F = Family relationships

   a) Family structure. Who is in the family? What are family member's roles? Roles of children, older adults, gender differences in roles. Who is the head of the household? Who takes care of children?

   b) Family dynamics. How does the family function and complete tasks. How are decisions made? Who manages finances? Is it important to have family present when someone is sick?

   c) What goals are important to family?

   d) Example. Asian families value and respect elders, children are expected to be loyal to the family and care for family members. African Americans have a strong family orientation, it is important for family to be present when someone is sick

5. H = Health and health beliefs

   a) Health beliefs refer to convictions that influence health behavior. What the person believes about health and the cause of health problems or disease

   b) Questions related to health beliefs include

      (1) What does the person do to stay healthy?

      (2) Who would they consult if they have a health problem?

      (3) How does the person explain illness? What causes illness? Some explanations include, a virus, something being out of balance, evil spirits, or a punishment from God

      (4) How does the person respond to health problems? Is the person stoic and tries not to show emotion? Or is the person expressive and openly displays emotions? For example, how does the person respond to pain? Does the person want analgesics? Do they believe that pain should be endured?

      (5) Examples of health and illness beliefs: Chinese Americans may believe that health and a happy life can be maintained if there is a balance between yin and yang. Heaven is yang; the earth is yin. The concept of qi, a vital force of life, is central to traditional Chinese medicine. The focus of health is having a healthy body, a healthy mind, and a healthy spirit. Chinese may use herbal therapy or acupuncture along with Western medicine. Many Chinese fear death and avoid talking about it

6. E = Education

   a) Education refers to a person's cognitive style and completion of a program of learning. Considerations include

      (1) How does the person learn best? Visual aids? Printed materials? By watching and doing?

      (2) How much formal education did the person complete? High school? Technical school? College? Degrees earned?

      (3) Occupation or profession

b) Examples: an older adult may learn best by doing, have less than a high school education, and be a successful owner of a business. A younger adult may learn best by audio-visual aids, have a college education, a bachelor's degree and be employed as a physical therapist

7. R = Religion

    a) Religious beliefs and practices

    b) Questions to consider

        (1) Does the person believe in God or gods?

        (2) What is the person's religious preference?

        (3) Does the person have any beliefs or practices that may have an impact on health and healthcare?

    c) Examples: Jehovah's Witnesses do not believe in blood transfusions. A Roman Catholic patient may want to have the Sacrament of the Sick. A Christian Scientist believes in spiritual healing and does not believe in using medications

V. **Culture and End of Life**[11-12]

A. **Dying and death are universal life experiences. Death is something we all experience, yet we know very little about it**

B. **Death systems of some type are found in every society.**[5,11-13] **Death system is defined as "the interpersonal, sociocultural, and symbolic network through which an individual's relationship to mortality is mediated by his or her society"**[13]

C. **A death system is made up of people, times, places, objects, and symbols. The death system in our culture seems to act to keep death at a distance. We avoid talking about death and our death system supports denial of death**

1. People: individuals have roles related to death (e.g., funeral director, life insurance agent, and florist)

2. Time: occasions associated with death (e.g., Good Friday, Memorial Day, the anniversary of a death)

3. Places: specific locations that have an association with death (e.g., a cemetery or funeral home)

4. Objects: things that are linked to death (e.g., a death certificate, tombstones, death notices in newspaper)

5. Objects or actions that signify death (e.g., a black armband, a skull and crossbones, certain organ music)

D. **Functions of a death system are to**

1. Give us warnings and predictions of danger (e.g., sirens, flashing lights)

2. Prevent death (e.g., police officers or emergency care personnel)

3. Care for the dying (e.g., a hospice)
4. Dispose of the dead (e.g., funeral industry)
5. Work toward social consolidation after death (e.g., work of funeral industry and cemeteries)
6. Make sense of death (e.g., religious systems)
7. Bring about socially sanctioned killing (e.g., capital punishment, training for war)

E. **September 11, 2001 and functions of death system**
1. Warnings not given priority, attack occurred without warning. Failed to prevent death on airplanes and ground. First responders reduced number of casualties
2. Caring for dying: many casualties occurred on the scene, emergency workers provided care. Many volunteers providing aid and assistance
3. Disposing of the dead: very long and stressful process
4. Social consolidation after death: delay in stress and grief for many families because bodies not found. American people responded with compassion
5. Making sense of death: major issue after unexpected deaths. Personal reflection of own death. Renewed sense of national unity. Many memorial services held
6. Killing: shift to war on terrorism after being victims of external death system

VI. Culture and End-of-Life Decision-Making[11-13]

A. **American cultural belief in self-determination and autonomy includes people making their own decisions about end-of-life care**

B. **People should be told the truth about their illness in order to make an informed decision**

C. **The passage (1991) of the Patient Self-Determination Act was based on widespread acceptance of belief that everyone should have an advance directive**
1. No studies have shown that advance directives facilitate end-of-life decision-making or guide care
2. The Study to Understand Prognoses and Preferences for Outcomes and Risk of Treatment[14] (SUPPORT) was a concentrated intervention study to improve shared decision-making in seriously ill adults. The intervention failed to make any improvements in patient involvement in end-of-life care and decision-making

D. **Many cultural groups in the United States may not share these views about autonomy and end-of-life decision-making**

E. **Older adults may believe the physician knows best and should be the decision-maker**

F. **Older adults may choose to defer to adult children to make decisions for them**

G. Some groups believe telling a person their prognosis is harmful because it takes away hope. Talking about death may make it happen

H. Persons with a disability are fearful of advance directives because they believe they would be denied care

I. Minority groups or people of color who have experienced discrimination in healthcare are fearful that signing an advance directive would mean no care

VII. Selected Multicultural Views of End-of-Life Decisions[11–13,15,16]

A. American Indians believe truth telling violates their tradition and talking about bad things makes them happen. Beliefs vary by tribal groups

B. African Americans are not likely to complete an advance directive. As a group they have experienced oppression and discrimination and would question why end-of-life care would be any different. The family usually makes decisions about healthcare

C. Asian Americans: the family is the primary decision-maker. Families are unlikely to tell a seriously ill person they are dying. They believe protecting someone from the truth allows him or her to have hope

D. Mexican Americans have a very strong family orientation. Family members bear the responsibility of hearing bad news and protecting the family member. Spiritual orientation is important and they want the family member to receive sacraments from a priest

E. Healthcare providers need to be careful about assuming all members of a group share the same beliefs and values about advance directives. It is important to learn about the individual patient's values

VIII. Culture and End-of-Life Symptom Management[5,12]

A. Responses to Pain

1. Culture influences responses to pain and the emotions people use to express pain

2. Some cultures allow open and free expression of pain; other cultures avoid the expression of emotions and pain

3. Gender may influence expression of pain. American males are socialized not to express emotions such as crying

B. Meaning of Pain

1. The word pain is derived from Greek word for penalty. Helps to explain the association between pain and punishment in Judeo-Christian thought

2. Pain is a part of life (e.g., Navajo consider pain a way of life)

3. Pain assessments should include the cultural meaning of pain

C. **Pain Management**

1. Majority of older adults in nursing homes have untreated or under treated pain. Many older adults believe pain is part of being old

2. Culture influences response to pain (e.g., facial expressions, requests for relief of pain, and verbalizations about pain)

3. Alternative and complementary therapies may be used to treat pain (e.g., acupuncture, relaxation techniques, yoga, and meditation). Ask clients what they use to decrease pain. What has been helpful?

D. **Nutrition**[17]

1. Food and liquids are essential to life and are associated with nurturing and comfort

2. Decisions about artificial nutrition and hydration are controversial. Some families believe that not providing food and fluids is inhumane and results in a painful death by starvation

3. Cultural groups may have beliefs specific to food and hydration

4. Artificial nutrition and hydration are not likely to promote comfort or enhance quality of life for most terminally ill patients

5. Nurses should provide families and clients with information on food and hydration so they can make an informed decision

IX. Cultural Responses to Death and Death Rituals[4,5,10,12,13]

A. **There is a serious lack of data on how ethnic minorities in the United States deal with dying, death and bereavement.[12,13] The majority of studies have been done with small samples**

B. **Need to be careful about stereotyping and assuming everyone is like the dominant culture in the United States. There is more variation in groups than between groups**

C. **Rituals associated with death are found in every society. Death rituals assist the individual and society with how to act in unfamiliar situations. They provide a meaning for a loss and function to restore social order. They provide a means for coping with loss. Funeral and memorial services contribute to making real the implications of death**

D. **Death rituals of religious, ethnic and cultural groups are the least likely to change over time**

E. Examples of rituals in American society include: the death of President, police officer, or member of the military is associated with a formal and elaborate funeral, burial, and memorial services. The funeral services for President Reagan are examples of rituals. They included the horse without a rider and the boots facing backwards. Other examples: firing a gun, playing "taps," roadside memorials placed where someone died, members of sports teams wearing black arm bands

F. Examples of cultural and religious variation in death rituals[4,5,10,12,13]

1. Orthodox Jews bury their deceased before sundown of the next day and have after-death rituals for several days[4]

2. Mexican Americans hold elaborate ceremonies, for example a *velorio* to honor the dead.[4] May express intense feelings of grief

3. In Asian American families the son may assume role of major decision-maker for the family. Less likely to tell seriously ill persons they are dying

4. African Americans have a strong religious and family orientation. It is important for family members to be present when someone is seriously ill. Openly express their emotions about the loss of a family member

5. American Indians view death as a natural process, favor having person die in a hospital so the home is not polluted by death

6. Hmong believe the person should be dressed in the finest traditional Hmong clothing so he or she will enter the next world well dressed

7. Muslims face Mecca when approaching death and recite passages from the Holy Qur'an

G. Healthcare providers should ask families if they have any practices that are important to them when someone dies. Avoid making assumptions about what families want. It may also be helpful to ask the family who is a spokesperson for the family

X. Cultural Response to Death: Grief and Mourning[4,5,10,12,13]

A. Grief is an affective response to a loss. Mourning is a culturally patterned response to loss[18]

B. Expressions of mourning differ among groups. Many people are reluctant to express their grief in public places such as a hospital

C. Grief is a universal phenomenon that is strongly influenced by culture

D. Bereavement is universal, however it's meaning to the individual varies cross-culturally

E. In American culture there is no clearly defined period of mourning. People are suppose to "get on with living"

F. **Other cultures have clearly defined periods of mourning and follow certain rituals**[4,5,10]

1. Chinese Americans' death and bereavement traditions are centered on ancestor worship. It is a form of paying respect. Belief that the spirits cannot rest until living relatives provide care for the grave and worship the memory of the deceased. The color white is associated with death and is bad luck

2. Orthodox Jews believe the dying person should not be left alone. Burial usually occurs 24 to 48 hours after death. Funeral service is directed toward honoring the departed. Shiva (Hebrew for seven) is the seven-day period that begins with burial. When mourners are "sitting Shiva" they do not work. Mirrors are covered to decrease the focus on one's appearance. The *kaddish*, a prayer for the dead, is said. Mourning for a parent lasts for one year

3. Mexican Americans are stoic and view death as a part of life. It is important for all family members to be present. Family gathers for a *velorio*, a festive watch over the body of the deceased person before the burial

XI. **Summary**

A. The United States is a culturally diverse society with people from many different cultural traditions. The population is continuing to be diverse as people are immigrating into the United States from many countries

B. Culture influences what people believe about death and dying, the places of care for the sick and who is consulted about health problems. Health practices are influenced by culture

C. Healthcare providers need to be culturally competent in order to provide care that is culturally appropriate and promotes death with dignity

D. The process of becoming culturally competent begins with you having the desire to do so. Examine your biases and beliefs. Ask questions and be willing to learn

E. Avoid making assumptions. There is variation in all groups and there is more variation within groups than between groups

F. Consider the guidelines presented here. Enjoy your journey to cultural competence!

CITED REFERENCES

1. Tylor EB. *Primitive Culture* (Vols. 1 & 2). London, UK: Murray; 1871.

2. Galanti G. *Caring for Patients from Different Cultures*. 4th ed. Philadelphia, PA: University of Pennsylvania Press; 2008.

3. Fong CM. Ethnicity and nursing practice. *Top Clin Nurs.* 1985;7(3):1–10.

4. Giger JM, Davidhizar RE, eds. *Transcultural Nursing: Assessment & Intervention*. 4th ed. St. Louis, MO: Mobsy, Inc.; 2004:3–19.

5. Purnell LD, Paulanka BJ. Transcultural diversity and health care. In: Purnell LD, Paulanka BJ, eds. *Transcultural Health Care: A Culturally Competent Approach*. 3rd ed. Philadelphia, PA: Davis; 2008:1–19.

6. Institute of Medicine (US). Committee on communication for Behavior Change in the 21st Century: Improving the health of diverse populations. *Speaking of Health: Assessing Health Communication Strategies for Diverse Populations*. Washington, DC: National Academies Press; 2002.

7. Quick Facts. U.S. Census Bureau. *People Quick Facts*. Derived from population data. 2007–2008. Available at: http://quickfacts.census.gov/qfd/states/00000.html. Accessed July 28, 2009.

8. Jenko M, Moffitt SR. Transcultural nursing principles: an application to hospice care. *Journal of Hospice and Palliative Nursing.* 2006;8(3):172–180.

9. Zoorenbos AZ, Schim SM. Cultural competence in hospice. *Am J of Hosp & Palliat Care.* 2004;21(1):28–32.

10. American Geriatrics Society, Adler R, Kame H. *Doorway Thoughts: Cross-Cultural Health Care for Older Adults*. Boston, MA: Jones & Bartlett Publishers; 2004.

11. Corr CA, Nabe CM, Corr DM. *Death and Dying: Live and Living*. 6th ed. Belmont, CA: Thomson/Wadsworth; 2008.

12. Werth JL, Blevins D. *Decision-Making Near the End of Life: Issues, Developments, and Future Directions*. New York, NY: Routhlede; 2009.

13. Kastenbaum RJ. *Death, Society and Human Experience*. 10th ed. Upper Saddle River, NJ: Pearson Education, Inc.; 2008.

14. SUPPORT Principal Investigators. A controlled trail to improve care for seriously ill hospitalized patients. The study to understand prognoses and preferences for outcomes and risk of treatments (SUPPORT). *J Am Med Assoc* 1995;274:1591–1598.

15. Drought TS, Koening BA. "Choice" in end of life decision-making: research fact or fiction? *The Gerontologist*. 2002;42(Special Issue III):114–128.

16. Teno J, Lynn J, Wenger N, et al. Advance directives for seriously ill hospitalized patients: effectiveness with the Patient Self-Determination Act and the SUPPORT intervention. *J Am Geriatrics Society* 1997;45:500–507.

17. Ersek M. Artificial nutrition and hydration: clinical issues. *J Hosp Pallia Care*. 2003;5(4):221–230.

18. Andrews MM, Boyle JS, eds. *Transcultural Concepts in Nursing Care*. 5th ed. Philadelphia: Lippincott; 2008.

Additional References and Resources

Braun KL, Karel H, Zir A. Family response to end of life education: differences by ethnicity and stages of care giving. *Journal of Hospice and Palliative Medicine.* 2009;23(4):269–276.

Crawley LM. Racial, cultural, and ethnic factors influencing end of life care. *Journal of Palliative Medicine.* 2005:8(supplement 1):S58–S69.

Gutheil IA, Heyman JC. "They don't want to hear us." Hispanic elders and adult children speak about end of life planning. *Journal of Social Work in End of Life Care.* 2006;2(1):55–70.

Hayes C. Ethics and end of life. *Journal of Hospice and Palliative Nursing.* 2004;6(1):36–43.

Hussein A, Nijmeh M. Cultural diversity and cancer pain. *Journal of Hospice and Palliative Nursing.* 2009;11(3):154–164.

Ludke RL, Smucker DR. Racial differences in the willingness to use hospice services. *Journal of Palliative Medicine.* 2007;10(6):1329–1336.

Mancuso L. Proving culturally sensitive palliative care. *Nursing.* 2009;39(5):50–53.

Sutermaster DJ, Grandovic NL. *Cultural Impact on Managing Pain and Associated Side Effect.* Pittsburgh, PA: Hospice and Palliative Nurses Association; 2010.

Wilson SA, Coenen A, Doorrenbos A. Dignified dying as a nursing phenomenon in the United States. *Journal of Hospice and Palliative Nursing.* 2006;8(1):34–41.

Chapter VIII

Spiritual Care at the End of Life

Barbara Anderson Head, PhD, RN, CHPN®, ACSW

Adapted from: Head B. Spiritual care at the end of life. In: Ersek M, ed. *Core Curriculum for the Hospice and Palliative Nursing Assistant.* Dubuque, IA: Kendall Hunt Publishing; 2003:93–99.

I. **Definitions**

    A. **Definitions of Spiritual or Spirituality**[1-4]

        1. That part of the person, often known as the soul, which connects to a superior being, "higher power," or force such as God

        2. Awareness of a divine presence

        3. Person's sense of meaning or purpose in life

        4. "Harmonious relationships or connections with self, neighbor, nature, God, or a higher being that draws one beyond oneself"[4, p. 663]

        5. May include religious beliefs and practices, but does not require that one participate in organized religion

    B. **Aspects of Spirituality**

        1. Attributes of Spirituality[5-7]

            a) Meaning: finding the reason for what has happened in a person's life and what is happening now

            b) Value: what is cherished by the individual

            c) Transcendence: moving beyond oneself and the situation

            d) Connecting/Relatedness: connection or relationship with a higher being or faith community

            e) Becoming: reflecting on one's life that results in knowing who one is

            f) Hope: finding the good that could be

            g) Forgiveness: the need to pardon others or oneself for acts against us or others

C. **Definition of Spiritual Well-Being**
1. A sense of inner peace, compassion for others, reverence for life, gratitude, and appreciation of both unity and diversity[8]

D. **Definitions of Religion**
1. An organized effort to express one's spirituality often through rituals and specific practices such as prayer, communion, baptism, and meditation[7]
2. A particular way of expressing one's spirituality through certain beliefs and behaviors[9]

E. **Definitions of Spiritual Care[7]**
1. Any palliative care team member's response to the patient's spiritual needs through various interventions, such as listening, accepting, talking and being with the patient and family about life and its meaning, and coordinating care with the patient's religious community
2. Efforts to help the patient have a feeling of spiritual well-being
3. Providing opportunities for reconciliation or relationship with a higher power (such as God), self and others[7]

II. **Importance of Spiritual Care in Palliative Care**

A. **Spiritual beliefs affect how a person lives and dies**

B. **Spiritual beliefs affect the patient and family's acceptance of hospice/palliative care**

C. **Hospice/palliative care is holistic; it deals with the physical, social, psychological, and spiritual parts of the patient and family**

D. **Spirituality contributes to quality of life for the dying patient**

E. **Spiritual beliefs and practices help the patient and family cope with terminal illness**

III. **Spiritual Needs of the Dying Patient**

A. **Give and receive love**

B. **Give and receive forgiveness**

C. **Find meaning and purpose in one's life**

D. **Life review or telling the story of one's life**

E. **Develop hope that life can be lived fully and deeply**

F. Develop hope for a life after death

G. Finish unfinished tasks

H. Mend broken relationships

I. Have positive relationships with God and others

J. Find meaning with one's life, illness and dying

K. Participate in religious beliefs and practices (prayer, Bible reading, meditation)

L. Accept one's self and be at peace

M. Die with dignity

IV. Fears or Concerns of the Dying Patient Related to Spirituality

    A. Loss of control and dignity

    B. Loss of personal self

    C. Loss of family and friends

    D. End of life as we know it

    E. Lack of meaning in life and death

    F. Being a burden to others

    G. The unknown

    H. What happens after death

    I. Loneliness or dying alone

    J. Pain and other symptoms

V. Questions Patients Might Ask That Indicate a Spiritual Need or Concern

    A. Where is God?

    B. Why must I suffer?

C. Do you believe in God?

D. What do you think happens when we die?

E. Will you pray for me?

F. Why did I get this disease?

G. "Why" questions that do not depend upon technical answers are often spiritual in nature (Charles von Gunten)[10]

VI. Spiritual Signs That Death Is Coming Soon[11]

A. Lack of interest in material goods and things

B. Less interest in talking about things that are not really important

C. More silence

D. Lack of concern for appearance (how one looks)

E. Less interest in some relationships

VII. Common Religious/Spiritual Views on Death and Death Rituals[7,12,13]

A. The following information is general; not every member of each religion adheres to all practices and beliefs of a particular religion

B. Buddhist beliefs and practices

1. Focus of most Buddhist practices is to attain a calm state of mind and to be full of compassion
2. State of mind at the time of death is important: patient may refuse medications that cloud the mind
3. Illness is a result of actions in this world or a previous life
4. Healing results from knowing the wisdom of Buddha
5. A temple or altar with a statue of Buddha may be in the house
6. Frequent meditation or chanting
7. Death is viewed as part of life and offers the chance to improve in the next life
8. It is important to assist the dying to let go
9. Some believe that the soul remains around the body for several days
10. Family may ask that body be untouched for as long as possible so the spirit can make a peaceful transition to the next world

C. **Roman Catholic beliefs and practice**
   1. Central focus is to obtain eternal life with God in heaven
   2. Illness may be viewed as punishment for sinful thinking or behavior
   3. Use of many signs or symbols such as the cross, the crucifix, holy water, statues of saints
   4. Important to attend Mass on Sunday and holy days
   5. Praying is very important, may involve praying the rosary
   6. The ill may receive the Sacrament of the Sick

D. **Hindu beliefs and practices**
   1. Death is natural and unavoidable, but is not actually real
   2. Death is seen as a pause in the eternal journey
   3. Do not eat beef, often practice fasting
   4. Physical modesty and cleanliness is very important
   5. Belief in many reincarnations before obtaining union with Brahman (God)
   6. Believe in four social classes (castes); person inherits his or her social class at birth
   7. Body is washed, anointed, and dressed in new clothes after death
   8. Body is cremated and water burial is preferred
   9. Only those of the same social class can touch the body
   10. Doing good deeds and giving to the needy are important

E. **Jewish beliefs and practices. Content here refers to Orthodox beliefs. There are different levels of observance: Orthodox, Conservative, Reform, Reconstructionist, and Unaffiliated that have varying beliefs and practices**
   1. Focus on life and preserving it
   2. Death is not to be feared as it is natural and comes from God
   3. Soul exists before the body and continues to live after the body is dead
   4. Kosher foods are eaten and should be made available. As per the Torah, Kosher refers to certain foods that can and cannot be eaten (e.g., pork is not permitted) and how foods are to be prepared (e.g., meats and dairy products must be eaten separately)[14]
   5. The Sabbath celebration starts on Friday at sunset to Saturday at sunset and certain activities may not be allowed
   6. After death the body is not left alone until burial
   7. Person's eyes should be closed immediately after death, preferably by the deceased person's children
   8. Dead body receives a special washing by the *Chevra Kadisha*, specially trained members of the Jewish community
   9. Burial within 24 hours (except no burials on the Sabbath)
   10. Death is followed by seven days of intensive family mourning; this period is called Shiva

F. **Muslim or Islamic beliefs and practices**
   1. Patient may want to use remaining time for prayer and meditation
   2. Patient may want to read from their holy book, the Qu'ran
   3. Members may follow strict dietary guidelines and period of fasting
   4. Five periods of prayer are required daily
   5. Patient will want to face east towards Mecca when praying
   6. Believe that peace follows total submission to the will of God
   7. Want the dying person to face death with calmness
   8. Death is considered a natural process and a return to God
   9. Cleanliness is important and may require bathing, cleaning at least five times per day before the required five periods of daily prayer; personal hygiene provided by persons of opposite gender may be very distressing
   10. Body must be turned to face Mecca (the holy city) at the time of death

G. **Protestant beliefs and practices**
   1. God is single being who spoke to people through the Bible
   2. God protects, judges, and forgives those who ask
   3. Believers have a direct and personal relationship with God
   4. Focus on salvation through the gift of God's grace in Jesus' death
   5. Belief in afterlife, heaven is promised based on personal salvation

VIII. Spiritual Interventions (Actions) of the Licensed Practical/Vocational Nurse

A. **Reasons for the licensed practical/vocational nurse to provide spiritual care**[15]
   1. Spiritual needs may surface at any time and are best cared for if addressed immediately
   2. Spiritual care needs do not occur separate from other care needs or only when a chaplain is present
   3. Spiritual caregiving requires a trusting relationship such as often occurs between the patient and the nurse

B. **Be a good listener**
   1. Allow the patient and family to express their feelings
   2. Do not rush the patient or family when they want to talk
   3. Ask questions to encourage patient and family to talk about their beliefs, or lack of beliefs, but do not make judgments about what they say
   4. Allow periods of silence and acceptance

C. **Develop a trusting relationship with the patient and family**

1. Show an interest in patient's and family's feelings and beliefs
2. Be compassionate: let patient and family know you care about them
3. Remain present with the patient through periods of fear and suffering

D. **Be aware of suffering and the emotional pain of the patient**

1. Such suffering may include regrets, guilt, failures, anger, feeling alone
    a) Be aware that veterans, especially those who served during war, often experience spiritual distress for what they did, were not able to do, and/or saw during their service
2. Provide consistent, loving care
3. Report any physical or emotional pain to your other team members so the team can assist and intervene as needed

E. **Encourage and offer hope**

1. Patient's goals may change but they can still have hope
2. Patients can hope to live for a certain event or to complete a task
3. Patients can hope for the type of death they want

F. **Help the patient finish any unfinished tasks**

1. Talk to your team about any such tasks you identify
2. If team agrees, help with letter writing, making a phone call or allowing the patient to talk through a relationship that needs mending

G. **Encourage the presence of loved ones and a minister, rabbi or other spiritual leader**

H. **Assist the patient with life review**

1. Encourage the patient to talk about his/her life—special events, hobbies or interests, education, professional accomplishments, family
2. If patient has dementia, ask family members to share about the patient's life and what they were like before the illness
3. Notice and comment on photographs and mementos—ask the patient to talk about them

I. **Know the patient's plan of care related to spiritual issues**

1. If you have questions or concerns about the patient's spiritual needs or issues, talk to the team chaplain
2. Ask the chaplain how you can help with spiritual issues

IX. **Summary**

   A. **Spiritual care is the care provider's response to the patient's need to connect with a superior force or being and give meaning to life**

   B. **Spiritual beliefs and practices are important to hospice and palliative patients and families**

   C. **Spiritual needs of the dying patient include love, forgiveness, finding meaning and purpose in life, life review, acceptance, and peace**

   D. **The major religions have different beliefs and practices related to death and dying**

   E. **Spiritual care interventions of the nursing assistant include being a good listener, encouraging religious practices and life review, respecting the patient's and family's beliefs and religious practices, developing a trusting relationship, assisting with unfinished tasks and working with the team to plan and carry out spiritual care**

CITED REFERENCES

1. Taylor EJ. Spiritual assessment. In: Ferrell BR, Coyle N, eds. *Textbook of Palliative Nursing*. 2nd ed. New York, NY: Oxford University Press; 2006:581–594.

2. American Association of Colleges of Nursing and the City of Hope National Medical Center. Module 1: Nursing Care at the End of Life. *End-of-Life Nursing Education Consortium (ELNEC) Project*. 2009. Funded through the Robert Wood Johnson Foundation.

3. Speck P. Spiritual issues in palliative care. In: Doyle D, Hanks GWC, MacDonald N, eds. *Textbook of Palliative Care*. New York, NY: Oxford University Press; 1998:805–814.

4. Fehring RJ, Miller JF, Shaw C. Spiritual well-being, religiosity, hope, depression, and other mood states in elderly people coping with cancer. *Oncol Nurs Forum*. 1997;24:663–671.

5. Stephenson PL, Draucker CB, Martsolf DS. The experiences of spirituality in the lives of hospice patients. *Journal of Hospice and Palliative Nursing*. 2003;5(1):51–58.

6. Martsolf DS, Mickely JR. The concept of spirituality in nursing theories: differing world views and extent of focus. *J Adv Nurs*. 1998;27:294–303.

7. Kemp C. Spiritual care interventions. In: Ferrell BR, Coyne N, eds. *Textbook of Palliative Nursing*. 2nd ed. New York, NY: Oxford University Press; 2006:595–604.

8. Vaughn F. *The Inward Arc: Healing and Wholeness in Psychotherapy and Spirituality*. Boston, MA: New Science Library; 1986.

9. Altilio T, Indelicato RA, Eighmy J, Nahman E. Care of the patient and family. In: Berry PH, ed. *Core Curriculum for the Generalist Hospice and Palliative Nurse*. 2nd ed. Dubuque, IA: Kendall Hunt Publishing; 2005:147–168.

10. Hallenbeck JL. *Palliative Care Perspectives*. New York, NY: Oxford University Press; 2003:151.

11. Kalina K. *Midwife for Souls: Spiritual Care for the Dying*. Boston, MA: St. Paul Books and Media; 2007.

12. Kemp C. *Terminal Illness: A Guide to Nursing Care*. Philadelphia, PA: J.B. Lippincott; 1995.

13. American Association of Colleges of Nursing and the City of Hope National Medical Center. Module 4: Cultural considerations in end-of-life care. *End-of-Life Nursing Education Consortium (ELNEC) Project*. 2009. Funded through the Robert Wood Johnson Foundation.

14. *Kashrut: Jewish Dietary Laws*. Available at: www.jewfaq.org/kashrut.htm. Accessed February 8, 2010.

15. Taylor EJ. Spirituality and the cancer experience. In: Carroll-Johnson RM, Gorman LM, Bush NJ, eds. *Psychosocial Nursing Care along the Cancer Continuum*. 2nd ed. Pittsburgh, PA: Oncology Nursing Press; 2006:120–122.

Additional References and Resources

Belcher A, Griffiths M. The spiritual care perspectives and practices of hospice nurses. *Journal of Hospice and Palliative Nursing*. 2005;7(5):271–279.

Buck HG, McMillan SC. The unmet spiritual needs of caregivers of patients with advanced cancer. *Journal of Hospice and Palliative Nursing*. 2008;10(2):91–99.

Campbell CL, Ash CR. Keeping faith. *Journal of Hospice and Palliative Nursing*. 2007;9(1):31–41.

Hasty C, Shattell M. "Putting Feet to What We Pray About": The Experience of Caring by Faith-Based Care Team Members. *Journal of Hospice and Palliative Nursing*. 2005;7(5):255–262.

Kruse BG, Ruder S, Martin L. Spirituality and coping at the end of life. *Journal of Hospice and Palliative Nursing*. 2007;9(6):296–304.

Puchalski, CM. Spirituality and end-of-life care: a time for listening and caring. *Journal of Palliative Medicine*. 2002;5(2):289–294.

Sherman DW. Spiritually and culturally competent palliative care. In: Matzo ML, Sherman DW, eds. *Palliative Care Nursing: Quality Care to the End of Life*. New York, NY: Springer Publishing Co; 2001:3–22.

Sutermaster DJ, Grandovic NL. *Cultural Impact on Managing Pain and Associated Side Effects*. Pittsburgh, PA: Hospice and Palliative Nurses Association; 2010.

Urbansky D, Webb G. *Cultural Diversity in America: How Different Cultures Approach End-of-Life Issues*. Louisville, KY: Alliance of Community Hospices and Palliative Care Services, Inc; 2001.

Wayman LM, Gaydos H, Barbato L. Self-transcending through suffering. *Journal of Hospice and Palliative Nursing*. 2005;7(5):263–270.

Zen Hospice Project [website]. Available at: www.zenhospice.org.

Chapter IX

End-of-Life Care for the Child and Family

Christy Torkildson, RN, PHN, MSN

I. **Introduction**

    A. This section is intended to assist licensed practical/vocational nurses with a practical reference and guideline for caring for infants, children, and adolescents with life-limiting and progressive illnesses

    B. Guidelines are based on the age, developmental level, diagnosis, and family specific needs and goals. Guidelines also follow the *Standards of Practice for Pediatric Palliative Care and Hospice* and the *Clinical Practice Guidelines for Quality Palliative Care* (2nd ed.)[1,2]

    C. The range of illnesses, conditions, and developmental levels of these children and their families cross a wide spectrum too involved for this section. A generalized approach is offered that can be applied or modified for all children and their families; however some specific information about the most common pediatric life-threatening conditions is included

II. **Common Pediatric Diagnoses Seen in Palliative and Hospice Care**

    A. Cancer[3]

        1. These diagnoses continue to be the #3 cause of death overall for children 0–19 years of age and the #1 cause of death overall for children with complex chronic conditions[4]

            a) Leukemia is the most common form of childhood cancer

                (1) 80% of all leukemia cases are acute lymphocytic leukemia (ALL), followed by acute myelogenous leukemia (AML)

                (2) Diagnosis is often difficult because symptoms are similar to those of normal childhood illnesses. Onset can be slow or rapid. Parents often sense something is wrong however they cannot pinpoint why

(3) The child's history may include: fever, bleeding, pain (often back, leg or joint pain), and symptoms of anemia (fatigue/weakness, irritability, pallor, dyspnea); symptoms of thrombocytopenia (petechiae, purpura, bruising easily with minimal trauma); gastrointestinal symptoms (anorexia, abdominal pain, occasional weight loss, upper abdomen enlargement usually due to enlargement of the spleen and liver); symptoms of leukostasis/WBC clumping (headache, blurred vision, and respiratory problems due to leukemic infiltration of CNS and lungs); infections (often lymph nodes are enlarged usually in the neck or groin area); generalized achiness[5]

(4) Management includes: following CBCs, serum electrolytes during treatment. Children may have fever, bleeding, infections, neurological status changes, gastrointestinal changes, pulmonary changes, and genitourinary changes (painless gonadal swelling may indicate gonadal infiltrate). Pain and anxiety are also common

(5) Needs: discussion with the patient and family about the goals of treatments, desires regarding transfusions (curative vs. palliative), the risk of acute bleeds. Desires about antibiotic therapies in the case of fever as well as discussions about other potential complications from the disease as noted above. Effective pain management for treatment of pain or discomfort

b) Osteosarcoma: most common bone tumor in children

(1) History may include: original painful lesion in long bone (may or may not be associated with soft tissue mass and/or local edema). Common symptoms include malaise, fatigue, fever, anorexia, weight loss, and pain. Metastasis can be indicated by respiratory symptoms/distress; pain/symptoms from other sites such as bone, pleura, kidney, brain, or pericardium

(2) Management: follow systems noted above; follow changes in weight, changes in pain, and fevers. Multidisciplinary approach for pain and symptom management works best. Treatment of the tumor includes aggressive chemotherapy as well as aggressive surgery with either amputation or limb-salvage procedures in an attempt to maintain normal function. Treatment or tumor progression may be associated with limited function

(3) Needs: discussion with the patient and family about the goal of treatments, the impact of treatment on quality of life and measures to enhance quality of life. Effective pain and symptom management is essential

c) Rhabdomyosarcoma: most common soft tissue cancer in children

(1) History varies with anatomic location of tumor and the presence and extent of metastases: metastatic spread is via the blood and lymphatic systems, and frequent sites of spread are lung, bone, bone marrow, brain, spinal cord, lymph nodes, liver, heart, and breast; early spread within the muscle of origin and to adjacent tissue is common

   i. If the tumor is orbital (eye) in origin, history may include: orbital invasion, ptosis, exophthalmos, cranial nerve involvement (especially nerves II, III, IV, and/or VI) may be present

ii. If origin is non-orbital, parameningeal sites history may include: nasal obstruction, sinusitis, epistaxis, local pain, hypernasal speech, serous otitis media with facial palsy and conduction hearing loss. If the affected site is the ear there may be mucopurulent or sanguineous drainage; extension into the meninges is common along with symptoms of increased intercranial pressure (ICP). Seizures and/or headaches may be present with increased intercranial pressure

(2) Management: follow systems noted above; follow changes in weight, changes in pain, and fevers. Multidisciplinary approach for pain and symptom management works best

(3) Needs: discussion with the patient and family about the goal of treatments, the impact of treatment on quality of life and measures to enhance quality of life. Effective pain and symptom management is essential

d) Wilms' tumor: is the 4th most common type of cancer in children, it is a solid tumor that develops from immature kidney cells known as nephroblastoma; a malignant embryonal neoplasm of kidney, typically diagnosed between 1–5 years

(1) History: a painless abdominal mass in an otherwise healthy child. Frequently hematuria, and hypertension are present. The patient may have symptoms related to metastatic sites (i.e., lung, liver, brain, bone). On rare occasions, Wilms' tumor arises in both kidneys either at the same time or later on in the disease process (synchronous or asynchronous primary tumors)

i. Most patients referred to palliative care or hospices are referred due to metastatic disease, not primary disease. Wilms' tumor is 90% curable if diagnosed before metastasis except in patients with an unfavorable cell type, which occurs in 25% of all Wilms' tumor patients

(2) Management: primary management is aimed at relief of symptoms, including pain. Renal insufficiency is a risk and must be monitored. Children may be eligible for kidney transplant but only if cancer free

(3) Needs: discussion with the patient and family about the goal of treatments, the impact of treatment on quality of life and measures to enhance quality of life

e) Neuroblastoma

(1) Origin: original mass is often found in the abdomen, adrenal gland, paraspinal ganglia, neck, paraspinal area of thorax, or pelvis. Metastasis, in order of usual occurrence, include bone marrow, bone, lymph nodes, liver, intracranial lesions from direct extension of bony sites in skull, skin, and testes

(2) History: pain, pathological fractures (high risk), abdominal masses which can include retroperitoneal lymph nodes; thoracic masses can induce superior vena cava (SVC) syndrome or Horner's syndrome (miosis, ptosis, exophthalmos, anhidrosis); paraspinal involvement may lead to spinal cord compression

(3) Unique issues: tumor progression and treatment often affect normal functioning. Outcomes have improved for children with lower stage of disease and overall outcomes have improved due to better patient stratification (i.e., better identification of low, moderate, and high-risk patients), which in turn means more accurate treatment for the stage of the disease. As in most cancers the higher the stage the worse the prognosis. Stage 4 disease had a probability of an event free survival of only 25% and now it is approximately 40%. Overall children with cancer have improved survival of their primary disease however secondary cancers and co-morbidities due to the aggressive treatment remain challenging

(4) Needs: discussion with the patient and family about the goal of treatments, the impact of treatment on quality of life and measures to enhance quality of life

f) Brain tumors

(1) Signs and symptoms prior to diagnosis may include: irritability, lethargy, vomiting, anorexia, headache, papilledema, behavioral changes (i.e., problems in school), gross motor difficulties (i.e., increased falling, changes in ability to walk), seizures, bulging fontanels in an infant. Signs and symptoms of pending herniation may appear if early signs of a brain tumor are not recognized. These include: changes in vital signs (including widening of pulse pressure, bradycardia, and respiratory irregularity)

(2) Signs and symptoms with disease progression may include: increased frequency or severity of all symptoms noted above, decreased level of consciousness, loss of sensation, decrease in voluntary movement, difficulty in swallowing, malnutrition, and dehydration. Side effects of therapy may lead to bleeding and changes in self-esteem due to change in appearance (often due to Cushing's syndrome from large doses of steroids)

2. Spectrum of cancer in children differs markedly from that in adults

a) Childhood cancer: usually involves hematopoietic system, nervous system, and connective tissue

b) The following rarely occur in adults: neuroblastoma, Wilms' tumor, retinoblastoma, and hepatoblastoma[6]

B. Non-Cancer Diagnoses

1. Congenital anomalies

a) Two major types of congenital anomalies

(1) Malformations, arising during embryogenesis (*the development and growth of an embryo, especially the period from the second week through the eighth week following conception*) such as anencephaly

(2) Deformations, late changes in previously normal structures due to pathologic processes or intrauterine forces (e.g., infections, hydrocephalus)

b) These anomalies account for the 3rd highest cause of death in children 0–14 and create the largest group of children who could benefit from a hospice or palliative care program. They include

(1) Trisomies such as 13 and 18; lower number trisomy most often are associated with stillbirths

(2) Osteogenesis Imperfecta Type II

(3) Cerebral dysgenesis such as anencephaly, holoprosencephaly and lissencephaly

(4) Cardiac anomalies not compatible with life or determined to be inoperable

c) Other conditions/pathophysiology appropriate for pediatric palliative care

(1) Progressive muscular diseases include muscular dystrophy. Muscular dystrophy includes a large number of conditions that involve progressive loss of muscle strength and voluntary movement compromising the respiratory system as the disease progresses

   i. Duchenne's muscular dystrophy is seen in boys often presenting in early childhood, with few patients surviving past the early 20s. This is an x-linked recessive disorder

   ii. Walker-Warburg syndrome is the most severe form of childhood muscular dystrophy with most children dying before 3 years of age. Clinical manifestations are usually present at birth and include hypotonia, developmental delay, mental retardation and seizures

d) Progressive neurological conditions include spinal muscular atrophy (SMA) where the nerves that enervate the muscles die off resulting in respiratory compromise and loss of voluntary movement. SMA classification has four groups in order of decreasing clinical severity. SMA I and SMA II are the conditions most likely to benefit from palliative and hospice care

(1) SMA I also known as Werdnig Hoffman Disease. This condition usually presents in the infant between 0–6 months of age and is the most severe form of the disease. Babies with SMA I generally do live beyond one year of life

(2) SMA II usually presents between 7–18 months of age. Infants tend to lose gross motor skills as the disease progresses. Children with SMA II lose gross motor skills as the disease progresses however life expectancy varies with each child. All children are not expected to survive childhood

e) Children who have been profoundly injured or had a sudden acute illness event and will not have life support continued for prolonged periods should be identified for hospice consultation and support

f) Hypoxic ischemic encephalopathy (HIE) which is often due to intrauterine or birth related trauma/events are also appropriate for early referral to pediatric palliative care

g) Other relevant conditions include metabolic/mitochondrial disorders such as: Tay Sachs, Menkes Syndrome

C. Perinatal Hospice

1. A prenatal diagnosis of a potentially lethal condition can be the catalyst for a hospice referral to support the expectant parents and other family throughout the pregnancy, labor and delivery

2. "Traditional" hospice support and care for the baby if he/she survives the immediate time of delivery

3. Grief support in anticipation of the possibility of death and bereavement support for the family when the baby dies and afterwards

4. Includes the same preventative approach to minimize physical, emotional and spiritual suffering and to prevent the initiation of unintended, undesired, or futile interventions; emphasis is on *Quality of Life* and creating opportunities for a personalized, family centered experience, regardless of the duration of the baby's life

III. Differences between Pediatric and Adult Hospice Care

A. Pediatric Issues[7]

1. Not legally able to make decisions regarding treatment; yet want to participate in decisions; assent versus consent

2. The child's needs may be perceived differently by parents than by the sick child or staff thus affecting provision of care and communication

3. May not have the verbal skills to adequately express feelings and needs

4. Have varied conceptions of and reactions to illness and death based on the following factors: age, developmental level; family/religious/cultural norms; cognitive, intellectual and emotional maturity

5. Has not achieved a "full and complete life"

6. Desire a sense of "normalcy" and typically prefer to be at home versus hospital

B. Family Issues[8]

1. Family is defined BY the patient and immediate caregivers/parents/guardians

2. Financial stressors: one or both parents may need to keep working, resulting in an inadequate support system

3. Respite often needed from being around-the-clock caregivers

4. Parents and staff must deal with sibling's feelings, which may include: acting out, anger, regressive behavior, anticipatory grief, fear, and/or problems at school

5. Fear of being alone and/or feelings of helplessness with responsibility of caring for their dying child

6. Adults often feel the need to protect the sick child and/or siblings by withholding information regarding diagnosis, treatment, and/or prognosis

7. Parental belief that "there must be something more that can be done"

C. Community/Agency Issues[8]

1. Must provide ongoing staff support and education regarding staff's own grief and personal issues

2. Lack of referrals from physicians hesitant to stop "curative" treatment, who may believe they have "failed the child and family"

3. Reimbursement for pediatric hospice care may be difficult to obtain and can be more costly than adult care

4. Assessment of "hospice appropriateness" of 6 months or less may be difficult to determine

5. Need ongoing commitment of agency to pediatric program in spite of small pediatric hospice population

D. **Staff Issues**[8]

1. Must be knowledgeable regarding physical assessment, pain and symptom management for infants and children, and pediatric disease processes

2. Staff may project fears for own children onto pediatric patient and family (i.e., "If it were my child . . ."; "They should . . .")

3. Must be able to recognize developmental level of child regarding cognitive understanding about death and dying

4. Need education on the real needs of dying children (i.e., children feel pain, want honest information and worry about their condition and its effects on others); be able to focus on "the living" yet to be done within the context of the child's limitations

IV. General Issues Related to Admission of Pediatric Patients

A. **Family-Centered Approach to Care**

1. Requires an interdisciplinary, collaborative team approach that focuses first and foremost on the needs of the *whole* FAMILY as a unit, to enable them to optimally thrive and cope within the context of the child's condition as it changes over time

2. Creates an inclusive model that optimally benefits the family and child, as the team works together to meet *their* goals for care and for *living*

   a) May include anticipatory grief support as well as bereavement support for the child and family with careful attention to the siblings

3. Typically requires a broader scope of individuals and providers, beyond the "patient/caregiver" model for adult hospice care

   a) *Whole* family care involves support and intervention for all of the family as the needs arise. May include the child's school as indicated or that of the sibling(s)

   b) May include child life specialist, multiple medical specialists, and ancillary staff such as PT, OT, play therapy, music, or art therapy, etc.

4. Sets a standard of involving the siblings in ongoing discussions and supports helping them understand the child's condition and clarify their perceptions of cause and expression of fears and concerns

   a) Siblings need to be included in the circle of care and their individual emotional, developmental, and basic needs met throughout the illness and into bereavement

   b) Feeling validated and supported during the sibling's illness and offering ways for the child to participate in the experience may assist him/her in adaptation during the illness and after child's death

B. **Identify Existing Support Systems**
   1. Determine what is available and also what is needed for the ill child's and/or sibling's school community as the child enrolls in hospice/palliative care and as condition progresses through child's death
   2. Collaborate with the social worker to maintain contact with child's school, identify mechanisms for classmate contact (counselor, teacher, etc.)
   3. Identify all who are directly contributing to the child's plan of care; may be multiple sites or providers such as multiple healthcare providers, home care agency and often several case managers. This also includes the family
   4. Identify existing spiritual and/or religious influences, beliefs, and supports for the child, siblings and parents belief system

C. **Treatment/Intervention Goals**
   1. Discuss with child's primary doctor and parents (and child as developmentally appropriate/physically capable)
      a) Goals for treatment therapies
      b) Goals that each person has, including the child to the extent possible based on developmental/cognitive level and parents wishes
      c) Use each change in condition or new symptom as an opportunity to review child and family goals
   2. Discussion of treatment options and goals for care is essential. Discussion to clarify as much as possible, the intent, benefit, burden, and *meaning* of the treatments for all involved is critical to a comprehensive plan of care made in concert with the child, family, and healthcare providers
   3. Upon discussion it may become evident that the understanding and perceptions of the goals of treatments may be shared, divergent, or conflicting among those involved
      a) Some interventions may be considered for continuation
      b) Others may be "titrated" down in intensity
      c) Other interventions may not be consistent with mutually agreed upon goals nor are contributing to quality of life for the child
   4. When creating a plan of care with the child and family, it is very important to place emphasis on the child's (as developmentally appropriate) and parent's *desired intensity of care* and symptom management for the child
      a) This requires a thoughtful, planned discussion with consideration of timing and the readiness of the child and parents to determine the depth of the discussion (i.e., is it time to discuss withholding or withdrawal or should that be another discussion and the first discussion is about current pain and symptom management alone)
      b) Key caregivers must participate
      c) Provide an appropriate setting for the discussion
      d) Be sure that adequate information is available, however caution must be exercised to prevent information overload for caregivers

D. Pain and Symptom Management: this section specifically highlights those distinctly different issues related to children and suggestions for helpful approaches

1. Thoroughly assess medical, psychosocial, spiritual needs and issues of the sick child, parents, siblings, and even grandparents OR EXTENDED FAMILY when involved directly with the care of the child

2. QUESTT[7]

    a) Q = Question the child. Verbal statement or description of pain is most important factor in pain assessment

    b) U = Use pain rating scales. Provides subjective quantitative measure of pain intensity

    c) E = Evaluate behavior. Common indicators of pain in children and are especially valuable in assessing pain in non-verbal children, including infants

    d) S = Secure parents' involvement because they know their child best

    e) T = Take cause of pain into account because pathology or procedure may give clues to expected intensity and type of pain

    f) T = Take action to meet the established goal (child's acceptable pain level) because the only reason to assess pain is to be able to relieve it through use of analgesic/adjuvant drugs and/or non-pharmacological methods

3. GOLDEN RULE: Whatever is painful to an adult is painful to a child or an infant!

4. Utilize a topical analgesic for blood draws or IV insertions to decrease fears or distress

5. Detailed guides for pain and symptom management in hospice and palliative care are found in other chapters in this book

6. Safe and effective pain management is essential regardless of age and size of infant or child

    a) As with adults' dosage guidelines are just that—guidelines. We treat the symptom or pain intensity not the numbers; however careful attention should be given to assessment for signs of any deleterious side effects. In addition, as with the adult attention must also be given to co-morbidities (i.e., is there renal impairment due to gestational age in a premature infant or to progressive disease or secondary to aggressive treatment that will affect the half-life or excretion of a particular medication)

    b) Acetaminophen (Tylenol®) use must be monitored and used sparingly as more evidence has shown the deleterious effects to the liver in patients of all ages[9,10]

    c) Never use aspirin or aspirin-containing medications for anyone 18 years old or younger

E. After-Hours Coverage and Continuity of Care

1. Needs of child/family should be assessed prior to admission to either hospice or palliative care program

    a) Consider if and how the individual hospice/palliative care program can meet anticipated needs

    b) If needs cannot safely and realistically be met with the present resources, identify additional or alternative resources in the community best equipped to handle and meet the pediatric patient/family needs

c) Attempt to create a collaborative framework to meet the needs of patient and family with all providers involved with child's care/family needs

2. For children and their families, a high priority must be placed on continuity of care

   a) Fragmented or poorly coordinated care for the child and family can exacerbate an already strained coping pattern

      (1) The nurse can facilitate communication between the providers and the family in order to maintain the established plan of care for the child/family and to avoid frustration, confusion and duplication of efforts

      (2) Maximizing opportunities to communicate between providers and ensure continuity between settings (home, clinic, hospital, school, etc.) is an important and primary role of the nurse

   b) As a "case manager" the nurse can keep the team and other healthcare providers updated on the evolving plan of care for the child and keep the existing support system intact for the benefit of the family

   c) Regular reports to referral sources can maintain optimal contact with the child's care team

V. Developmental Considerations in Pediatric Assessment

A. Special considerations for examining and interpreting assessment information are necessary for clinicians dealing with infants and children[11,12]

B. Appraisal of the child's developmental level is the first step toward a positive interaction, which reinforces the child's sense of security, mastery and self-esteem

1. Infant (0–1 year)

   a) Stranger anxiety is prevalent at 7 months of age and older; do physical examination with parent holding baby or within close view; smile; approach should be unhurried and gentle, use soft voice; avoid abrupt jerky movements

   b) Pain related behaviors: increased irritability, changes in crying patterns, handling/feeding changes, usual comfort measures less effective, facial expression is vigilant or angry, withdraws affected body part

      (1) In the first few months there is no apparent "understanding" of pain but baby has response to painful stimuli. *After repeated painful experiences even the youngest infant learns to fear pain*

      (2) Children develop anticipatory fear related to perceived painful situations, and as verbal skills develop use descriptive words for pain such as "owie, boo-boo, ouchie"

      (3) Ask parent/child how pain/hurt is referred to: utilize the familiar words for pain in the family; plan supportive interventions with parents; child may withdraw from social or play activity if pain persists[11,12]

2. Toddler (1–3 years)

   a) Separation and stranger anxiety starts to decrease

   b) Examine child in parent's lap, complete physical assessment through playful interactions (i.e., "Simon Says. . . ." or puppet play) and minimize initial physical contact

   c) Praise for cooperative behavior

   d) Identify words used for pain and discomfort

   e) Offer choices when appropriate

3. Preschool Child (3–5 years)

   a) Likes being a "helper," having choices and trying out equipment for him/herself

   b) Examine with parent close by

   c) Needs positive reinforcement and praise

   d) Less tentative than toddlers although may still have some stranger anxiety

   e) Identify words used by child to describe pain

   f) Offer choices when appropriate and incorporate measures that the child believes will work (i.e., what has been done at home, what they have seen). This can be the first step to including the child in the decision-making process

4. School-Age Child (5 years+)

   a) Able to understand simple explanations regarding illness and body functioning

   b) Developing understanding of "cause and effect," understands relationship between pain, other symptoms and disease process

   c) Provide age appropriate information and teaching regarding pain regiment and rationale

   d) Answer questions briefly and honestly

   e) Include child in decision-making process when possible

   f) Identify words to describe pain used by child

   g) Utilize dolls for "parallel" assessment and intervention

   h) Use appropriate picture books for aiding in explanation of bodily functions or changes

   i) Offer choices when appropriate and incorporate measures that the child believes will work

5. Adolescent

   a) More privacy and independence needed, prefers and should be included in explanation/findings

   b) More introspective; increasing use of mental/cognitive coping strategies; has capacity for coherent understanding of physiologic processes

   c) Allow for adolescent's input, insight, and choices

d) Attention needs to be given to self-esteem and personal image as it changes over time and is often related to peers. Develop strategies to decrease distress in this area, reinforce the positives and choices available

e) Participation in decision-making may be influenced by culture, age, and religious norms of family

VI. General Care Issues for Child/Family

A. Symptom Management Approaches

1. Nurse needs to be familiar with the child's developmental level to engage in any discussion on how they are physically feeling, for teaching related to care or disease progression, and selection of pain assessment tools

2. Give child and parent's choices in planning medication, treatments or procedures, and their daily living regimen to fit family lifestyle and goals for comfort

3. An important element of care for children and their families is the maintenance of NORMALCY in as many areas of life as possible and the incorporation of attention to physical appearance/self-esteem into daily routines

4. CONTROL is a most important aspect of approaching care for both the child and the parents

   a) The sick child may demonstrate an increased need for structure and routine as their scope of control diminishes

   b) This is normal and should be accommodated with an ongoing attempt to give choices and respect their need for routine that reinforces a sense of safety and security

5. Nursing visits typically involve some socialization activities with the child and siblings to create a therapeutic and relaxed environment prior to doing physical exam as a means of transitioning focus of time together

   a) Child will be more at ease when related to as a person first and as a sick child last

   b) Incorporate play into methods of communication as age appropriate

   c) Assume a relaxed posture, try to sit at child's level; avoid trying too hard which can come across as patronizing and *fake*

B. Planning Care for the Pediatric Patient

1. This patient population requires familiarity with and a planned response to any potential symptoms for the child's disease process and diagnosis

2. Identify those symptoms or perceived "emergencies" which the child and parents fear most and have a plan in place to respond quickly to treat them across possible settings (home, hospital, school, palliative care unit, inpatient hospice)

3. Nurses need to anticipate and prepare a plan for these to prevent and minimize experience of suffering fear of pain

4. Examples may include

a) Seizure management: have necessary medications in appropriate routes on hand for children with any neurological component to their disease to respond to any possible seizure symptoms, which may cause physical or emotional distress (suggestions include: lorazepam, gabapentin, phenobarbital, phenytoin, diazepam)

b) Pain management is essential for **all** ages

(1) Select appropriate routes and dosages *based on weight* (*mg/kg*) for infants and children

(2) Discuss with and provide education to parents and child on safe use, benefits of narcotics/opioids for pain relief and what to expect

   i. Assist them to create a schedule that fits their lifestyle and maintains desired level of relief

   ii. Consider cultural and ethnic influences as well as the exposure to education in schools related to illegal drug use (DARE programs, etc), which may influence perception of the use of therapeutic medications

(3) Consider combined strategies and/or methods for complex pain and multiple types of pain

(4) Assess for pain in the non-verbal child with behavioral indicators and facial expressions, appropriate pain assessment tools. Examples include[4]

   i. Poker chip tool (how many pieces of pain do you have?)

   ii. Eland color tool (selection of colors to represent intensity of pain applied to outline image of child's body)

   iii. Faces scale (series of 5 faces to represent range of pain ratings); numeric scales (usually 1–5 or 1–10)

(5) Pain in children can be approached with the principles of the WHO ladder as it applies to all patients

   i. The WHO Pain Ladder provides a treatment algorithm that recommends a step-wise approach to alleviating persistent pain. Each progressive step on the ladder represents medications with higher potency for increased severity of pain. These medications can be added to the patient's current medication or used instead of the current medication. The first step involves the use of mild analgesics. As with all pharmacological management of pain and symptoms, careful assessment of the child must be done to ascertain the best regimen for the child and family in conjunction with the physician or advanced practice nurse overseeing the child's care[13]

c) Anxiety and agitation

(1) Minimizing stress and anxiety in the child helps to reduce the suffering and anxiety of parents as well

(2) Agitation may arise related to tests and procedures, strangers, previous experience, untreated/under treated pain, and from fears related to his/her condition, one's future, concerns for self or family; fear of the unknown such as what will happen as they are dying, etc.

(3) Pharmacologic and non-pharmacologic interventions should be used such as relaxation/soothing strategies; reassess pain regimen for efficacy

d) Respiratory difficulties, dyspnea, congestion

(1) These can be very distressful to caregivers/parents and cause restlessness in the child

(2) Using medication to decrease secretions may benefit the child (glycopyrrolate, scopolamine, or atropine)

(3) Assess fluid intake versus volume tolerated

i. May need to adjust feedings if congestion continues

ii. Parents may need education on the symptoms of fluid overload, the inability to tolerate routine feedings in the child's current condition

iii. Gradually decreasing fluids based on demand and tolerance is easier for parents than an all-or-none approach

iv. Trial use of oxygen may be beneficial if it does not increase agitation (use pediatric nasal cannula, mask or blow by)

e) Elimination

(1) Maintain bowel function and prevent the acute stress and distress associated with constipation and the need for invasive remedies

(2) Invasive efforts to relieve constipation are very traumatic and risky for the child especially the oncology patient with bleeding precautions

(3) PREVENTION is very important via nutrition, hydration, and a preventative bowel regimen to avoid painful stooling/constipation. Hydration as long as possible to maintain urination, avoid indwelling catheters and maintain general comfort and hygiene

f) Blood products/transfusions

(1) Pediatric patients often benefit from continuing intermittent transfusions if they add to or maintain a desired quality of life; transfusions may help the child to accomplish specific personal goals (i.e., graduation, birthday, significant outing, or other milestone)

(2) These interventions may prevent a traumatic dying experience if it is expected that the child may actually hemorrhage or will die at home with that possibility

(3) There is constant need to plan ahead and include discussions of the balance of benefit versus burden for these therapies. The decision whether or not to provide them should not come as a surprise to the child or family. Reviewing the need for these therapies along with the benefit vs. burden and goals of care over time is also essential as the child's condition changes and the disease or condition progresses

g) Depression

(1) May not be anticipated but is not uncommon in the dying child or adolescent, and needs to be assessed PRIOR to symptoms appearing

(2) Children show the same symptoms as adults (i.e., becoming more withdrawn, apathy for known interests, decreased tolerance to change and increased labile emotions, irritability, sleep disorders, etc.)

(3) Consult with physician, social worker, psychologist or psychiatrist, to determine the best approach for each individual child

(4) Reassure parents and child that depression is treatable and not uncommon for both child and parents

(5) Utilize immediate onset medications for a more rapid therapeutic effect if indicated

C. **Preparation for the Last Days of Life**

1. Utilize hopeful language in context of condition; however do not set up unrealistic goals. Focus on the positive in the reality of the disease progression. For example, helping families with memory making (i.e., "making the most of 'Johnny's' time when he is awake as he will be sleeping more and more as the disease progresses")

    a) Negative and consistently "death oriented" discussions are not palatable, necessary, or wanted for most children and their families on a regular basis

       (1) Parents are often not prepared to make final arrangements until after the death

       (2) This may not be denial, but rather a personal decision reflecting the parents' needs and/or beliefs

    b) *Titrate* family's ability to handle these discussions, as trust and readiness are apparent

       (1) Forcing them may lead to conflict and hostility or even rejection of care

       (2) Hope is always present in some form and some expression for these families

2. As much as possible, plan where the death will take place

    a) With the help and support of the interdisciplinary team, discuss with patient and parents where they would prefer the death to occur

    b) Explore any fears or concerns—realistic or not—related to the decisions for place of death and dispel if appropriate

    c) Communicate the plan to all staff involved, especially those that cover after hours, at change of shift or assignments, etc.

3. Explore and discuss the spiritual dimension of the child's life as it relates to coping with their illness and life changes

    a) Have similar discussions with each parent and the sibling(s) and grandparents, if available

    b) Collaborate with chaplain/spiritual counselor to address the needs and concerns that arise during these discussions

       (1) Discuss what would bring comfort at this time and what continues to be a source of strength to each of them

       (2) Facilitate obtaining the desired spiritual and/or religious support

       (3) Provide for rituals requested

4. Prepare family members and child as he/she desires for what to expect as the dying process nears

   a) Providing this in a written form is particularly helpful for them to refer to and to use with other relatives

   b) Use language that is gentle, informative, and based on child's level of understanding

VII. Counsel/Provide Emotional Support for Child's Grief

A. Important to consider developmental stages as the context upon which to base explanations, education, needs assessment, and relevant approaches

1. If children have a sibling or a parent, significant grandparent, etc. who is dying, the issues of their grief need to be assessed and addressed by the interdisciplinary team (IDT)

2. IDT members, including the nurse, have significant opportunities to make the child feel included, to validate concerns and anticipatory grief, their desire to help and participate fulfilled—PRIOR to the death of their loved one

3. Grieving begins upon the realization something is seriously wrong or something has changed in the family. It does not wait for the knowledge that someone might be dying

B. Stages of Human Development—there are several theorists/theories; all believe that non-resolution of a particular stage may handicap a person in later life to some degree. Although this section is toward the end of this chapter the Stages of Human Development should be interwoven in ALL aspects of care for the child and family

1. Eric Erikson's Stages of Human Development: all stages are considered a "crisis that must be overcome and mastered"[14]

   a) Trust versus mistrust (infancy)

   b) Autonomy versus shame and doubt (early childhood)

   c) Initiative versus guilt (preschool)

   d) Industry versus inferiority (childhood)

   e) Identity versus diffusion (adolescence); directed toward dating and social roles

   f) Intimacy versus isolation (young adulthood)

   g) Generativity versus self-absorption (adulthood); most potential to change society

   h) Integrity versus despair (maturity)

2. Piagetian Stages[15,16]

   a) Sensory-motor (birth to 3 years): infant goes through several sub stages that lead from complete self involvement to learning through trial and error to use certain acts to affect an object or a person; by age 2, toddler learns that certain actions have a specific effect on the environment; thinking is egocentric (for instance, if mother leaves, child thinks it is because of his/her action)

b) Pre-operational (3–7 years): thought is intuitive and pre-logical (magical); thinking remains egocentric with conclusions based on what child feels or would like to believe

c) Concrete operational thought (7–12 years): conceptual organization becomes more stable and rational; child develops a conceptual framework that is used to evaluate and understand objects in the world around him/her

d) Formal operational thought (12–18 years): adolescent is increasing able to deal effectively with reality, abstract thinking, and future thinking; deductive reasoning develops; important ideals and attitudes develop in late adolescence

C. **Children and Grief Responses by Age** (*Note: children and adolescents do not grieve in a linear pattern but rather in a "clumping pattern" of sometimes intense periods separated by long intervals where they do not outwardly show that they are affected by the loss*)[12,17,18]

1. The infant: birth to 2 years (pre-verbal)

    a) Grief reactions: irritability, change in crying or eating patterns, bowel or bladder disturbances, emotional withdrawal, and slowing of development; clinginess; do not tolerate changes in daily living routine

    b) How to help: provide secure and stable environment, lots of TLC; follow a schedule, hold and play with the child often; a consistent caregiver and maintaining routines is critical

2. The preschool child: age 3–5 years

    a) Grief reactions: grasp of SOME concepts related to death, time and permanence are limited and often see death as temporary; may see seemingly inappropriate questions ("why cannot we just go out and get another brother?"), indifference, physiological symptoms (sleeping, eating, stomach aches), regression, fears, imagined guilt/feelings of responsibility, wide-ranging emotions

    b) How to help: same as above; understand and accept the behavior as normal; use the correct terminology; brief explanations; reassure the child he/she had nothing to do with causing the illness or death

3. The grade school child: age 6–10 years

    a) Grief reactions: a child of this age gradually begins to understand death, but may still believe that is only happens to other people; may feel guilt (magical thinking) and blame self for death; may see on-again, off-again grieving, problems in school (including socially inappropriate behavior, anger toward teacher or classmates, poor grades, physical ailments), anger; at this age children are at the most risk for complicated grief—they intellectually understand death, but lack coping skills to deal with the emotions

    b) How to help: same as above; provide simple, honest, and accurate information, accept behavior as normal, contact and ask for help from school counselors and teachers, acknowledge normalcy of anger and teach ways to constructively express it

4. The pre-adolescent and adolescent: age 10–18 years

   a) Grief reactions: typically, by age 12 to 14, children have a complete view of mortality; they may, however, deny that death can happen to them or one of their peers; may view death as punishment; grief at this developmental stage may interfere with the child's development of identity; may see hidden or denied emotions, so-called "common and normal adolescent behaviors" may be made worse by a loss at this stage (fighting, unruliness at school, rebellion, using drugs, sexual activity, suicidal tendencies)

   b) How to help: same as above; acknowledge that adolescents are not adults, and do not need to act or think like adults; evaluate supports available including at school; engage school and other trusted adults for support, be aware of destructive behaviors and set limits. Continue discipline parameters to maintain appropriate behavioral limits—this actually enhances security in the adolescent. Due to the inherent ambivalence and duality of feelings, intense emotions and desires for independence and tentativeness to release feelings; peer influences; may be interested in journaling, peer groups, tape recording, artistic expression, art therapy modes of expression

5. Young adult: age 19 and over

   a) Grief reactions: fully formed notion of death including how death affects him/her and changes in the family structure; may experience ambivalence and confusion about what is next for them, including the feeling of responsibility to take on some of the roles of the dead family member

   b) How to help: urge the young adult to focus on their needs and be able to express them to adults around them as well as peers so that others can support them; may be interested in support groups (not easy in the midst of the pain of grief!)

D. Ten Needs of Grieving Children[19]*

1. Adequate information

   a) Children need information that is clear and comprehensible

   b) When they do not have sufficient information, they'll make up a story to fill in the gaps

   c) If possible, children should be informed about an impending death; they already know something is taking place

   d) They can become anxious, maybe feel responsible, or may even wonder if they can *catch* whatever the cause of the person's death

2. Fears and anxieties addressed

   a) Children need to know they will be cared for; many children who lose one parent feel the other will die too; they fear for their own safety as well

   b) Children who lose a sibling fear they caused the death, that they will never be able to make it up to the parents or be "enough" for the parents

   c) Research has also shown that bereaved children who were given consistent discipline after a death were less anxious than those for whom discipline became lax

---

*Adapted by San Diego Hospice.

3. Reassurance they are not to blame

   a) Bereaved children of all ages may wonder, "Did I cause it to happen?" They need to know they did not cause or contribute to the death because of their anger or feelings

   b) Younger children may experience *magical thinking* which needs to be addressed with simplicity and truth at their developmental level

4. Careful listening

   a) Children need to have a person who will hear out their fears, fantasies, and questions and not minimize their concerns

   b) Some of their questions may be uncomfortable for adults, yet they need answers and validation. Encourage questions and ensure that they are treated with respect. It is okay to let children know you are uncomfortable, but not okay to brush off the question or their feelings

5. Validation of individual's feelings

   a) It is sometimes a temptation to tell a child how he or she should feel, but children's feelings must be acknowledged and respected as valid

   b) Children also need to express their thoughts and feelings in their own way

   c) Adults must remember each child's personality is unique as well as their relationship with the deceased

6. Help with overwhelming feelings

   a) Children need help in dealing with emotions that are too intense to be expressed

   b) The most common feelings expressed by bereaved children are sadness, anger, anxiety, and guilt

   c) Sometimes these feelings are acted out, and adults can help kids express them in safer ways through play activities and/or writing

7. Involvement and inclusion

   a) Children need to feel important and involved before the death as well as afterward

   b) For example, it is recommended that children over age 5 be allowed to make an informed decision as to whether or not they want to attend the funeral

   c) Children may want to have something special they have made buried with the person

   d) Children also need to be included in rituals around anniversaries or other special times when it's appropriate to remember the deceased in a more formal way

8. Continued routine activities

   a) Children need to maintain age appropriate interest and activities

   b) Adults sometimes need to be reminded that children cope and communicate through play activity (kids are kids first and grievers second)

9. Modeled grief behaviors

   a) Learning theory tells us that modeled behavior is one of the most effective sources of learning; children learn how to mourn by observing mourning behavior in adults

  b) Encouraging children to think about, to remember, and to talk about the deceased is a rather simple but effective way that adults can influence the course of bereavement in children

  c) Acknowledging and sharing feelings with the child in this way is very important

10. Opportunities to remember

  a) Children need to be able to remember and to memorialize their lost loved one not only after the death but also continuously as they go through the remaining stages of life

  b) Pictures and objects belonging to the deceased can be useful reminders of who the person was and the things that were important in the relationship; shared reminiscences can also be helpful

CITED REFERENCES

1. NHPCO. *Standards of Practice for Pediatric Palliative Care and Hospice, Children's Project on Palliative/Hospice Services (ChiPPS)*. Washington, DC: NHPCO; 2009:36.

2. National Consensus Project for Quality Palliative Care. *Clinical Practice Guidelines for Quality Palliative Care*. 2nd ed. Pittsburgh, PA: National Consensus Project for Quality Palliative Care; 2009: 90. Available at: www.nationalconsensusproject.org. Accessed February 8, 2010.

3. Goldman A. ABC's of palliative care: special problems of children. *BMJ*. 1998;316:49–52.

4. Friebert S. *NHPCO Facts and Figures: Pediatric palliative and hospice care in America*. Washington, DC: National Hospice and Palliative Care Organization; 2009.

5. Keene N. *Childhood Leukemia: A Guide for Families, Friends, and Caregivers*. 3rd ed. Sebastol, CA: O'Reilly & Associates, Inc.; 2002:1–13.

6. Children's Hospice International. *Children's Hospice International: 2001 Informational Overview*. Alexandria, VA: Children's Hospice International; 2001.

7. Wong DL. *Wong & Whaley's Clinical Manual of Pediatric Nursing*. 5th ed. St. Louis: Mosby; 2000.

8. Children's Hospice International. *Children's Hospice International: 2001 Informational Overview*. Alexandria, VA: Children's Hospice International; 2001.

9. Heubi JE, Barbacci MB, Zimmerman HJ. Therapeutic misadventures with acetaminophen: hepatotoxicity after multiple doses in children. *J Pediatr*. 1998;132(1):22–27.

10. Kubic A, Burda AM, Bockewitz E, Wahl M. Hepatotoxicity in an infant following supratherapeutic dosing of acetaminophen for twenty-four hours. *Semin Diagn Pathol*. 2009;26(1):7–9.

11. Clark E. *Palliative Pain and Symptom Management for Children and Adolescents*. Children's Hospice International and Division of Maternal and Child Health—U.S. Department of Health and Human Services: Alexandria, VA; 1985.

12. Huff SM, Hutton N. Pain and symptom management. In: Armstrong-Daily A, Zarbock S, eds. *Hospice Care for Children*. 3rd ed. New York, NY: Oxford University Press; 2009:24–53.

13. World Health Organization. *WHO's Pain Ladder*. 2010. Available at: www.who.int/cancer/palliative/painladder/en/. Accessed February 8, 2010.

14. Erikson E. *Childhood and Society*. New York, NY: W.W. Norton & Co.; 1963.

15. Wadsworth B. *Piaget's Theory of Cognitive Development*. New York, NY: David McKay Co.; 1971.

16. Petrillo M, Sanger S. *Emotional Care of Hospitalized Children: An Environmental Approach*. 2nd ed. Philadelphia, PA: J. B. Lippincott; 1980.

17. Volker B. *Hospice and Palliative Nurses Practice Review*. 3rd ed. Dubuque, IA: Kendall Hunt Publishing; 1999:96–97.

18. Gibbon MB. Psychosocial aspects of serious illness in childhood and adolescence: responding to the storm. In: Armstrong-Daily A, Zarbock S, eds. *Hospice Care for Children*. 3rd ed. New York, NY: Oxford University Press; 2009:54–75.

19. Worden JW. *Children and Grief: When a Parent Dies*. New York, NY: The Guilford Press; 1996.

CHAPTER X

FAMILY CAREGIVERS

Tami Borneman, RN, PHN, MSN, CNS, FPCN

I. Recognizing Roles/Needs of Family Caregivers at the End of Life[1-6]

    A. Terminal illness is a family experience

    B. Developmental stage of the family (e.g., teens, young adult singles, young parents with children, families with children in college, retired): individuals within the family unit respond differently to this experience and their relationship to the patient ultimately changes roles and functions as needed. These changes affect not only the individuals, themselves, but the family as a unit and ultimately the patient as well

        1. May influence type of response

        2. Will effect availability, especially during the working years

        3. Concerns and problems are different at different stages

        4. May affect availability of secondary caregiving support such as extended family

        5. Effects on family relationships

    C. Reduce physical and emotional burdens

    D. Provide family caregivers with knowledge and skill to enhance patient comfort, which will help reduce feelings of helplessness

    E. Provide resources for support

    F. Promote healthy coping

    G. Help prepare for the impending death

II. **Physical Concerns of Family Caregivers**[3,7-10]

   A. **Caregiving responsibilities concerning the patient**
      1. Administering medications
      2. Dealing with side effects of medication
      3. Providing help with or actually performing ADLs
      4. Wound dressing changes
      5. Managing ambulatory infusion pumps/other equipment
      6. Providing presence
      7. Providing symptom management (e.g., for pain, nausea, vomiting, shortness of breath, seizures, terminal agitation)
      8. Notifying the nurse when needed
      9. Shopping for needed items and picking up prescriptions

   B. **Physical concerns regarding their own person**
      1. Age of the family caregiver (many may be elderly)
      2. Fatigue
         a) Number of hours spent on caregiving/energy level
         b) Often only one family caregiver available, no other resources
      3. Sleep deprivation
         a) Caregiving is a 24 hour, 7 days per week job without any breaks
         b) Directly increases fatigue levels and impacts emotional well-being
      4. Chronic illness of their own, especially the elderly caregiver

   C. **Interventions**
      1. Provide resources for help in physical care and respite
      2. Use occupational therapists to teach work simplification and energy conservation skills
      3. Schedule a hospice aide to help with personal hygiene
      4. Assess caregiver's health status, chronic health problems and acute problems (e.g., fatigue, sleep deprivation, appetite)

III. **Emotional Needs of Family Caregivers**[1-3,5-6,11,12]

   A. **Help support, preserve, and/or develop emotions, thoughts and relationships with the patient and others**

   B. **Caregivers may recognize that they are in a stressful situation, they may not know how to alleviate and/or cope with the continued stress of caregiving**

C. **Specific emotional needs/issues**
   1. Anxiety
   2. Depression
   3. Fear
   4. Lack of connectedness
   5. Lack of knowledge about the disease and how to better care for their loved one
   6. Loss of control
   7. Perceived responsibility for relieving the patient's pain and suffering
   8. Uselessness
   9. Helplessness
   10. Anger/conflict
   11. Suffering from observing the patient's disease progression and physical decline

D. **Interventions**[1,3,7,13,14]
   1. Discuss concerns regarding future care
   2. Use psychiatric nurses and licensed clinical social workers
   3. Refer for respite care
   4. Facilitate sharing of feelings
   5. Assess for caregiver depression
   6. Help family members to *be* useful, not just to *feel* useful
   7. Help move the family's focus from cure to care
   8. Involve patient and family in care
   9. Help those involved to realize that anger is a normal response
   10. Help caregiver to fit tasks and helpers together and to be specific about what they need

IV. **Roles and Relationship Needs/Issues**[1–4,7,11,12,15]

   A. **Terminal illness impacts, to various degrees, the roles each member has performed**

   B. **Developmental stage of each member may affect coping with role changes**

   C. **Specific needs/issues**
      1. Perceived/actual lack of support from family and friends which can result in loneliness and isolation
      2. Anticipatory grieving can lead to anticipatory isolation

3. Loss of sexual intimacy
    a) Physical
    b) Emotional
        (1) Patient may not share feelings about this loss
        (2) Caregiver may not share emotions
        (3) Results of not sharing lead to further loneliness and isolation
4. Finances and employment
    a) Many times caregivers are having to work full or part time while also fulfilling caregiving responsibilities
    b) Expense of hiring help
    c) Financial depletion of savings/bankruptcy
    d) Some caregivers have to quit work
    e) Cost of health insurance premiums
5. Perceived inadequacies of services
    a) Can lead to feelings of abandonment
    b) Can lead to feeling unsupported not only professionally but socially as well

D. **Interventions**
    1. Minimize isolation and loneliness through available resources/networking
    2. Encourage when possible, sharing with each other or with a professional, concerns about sexual intimacy
    3. Utilization of hospice volunteers
    4. Meet with family members/friends to address personal concerns and to create realistic schedules for sharing caregiving duties
    5. Validate caregiver feelings about the burdens of caregiving and encourage them in what they are already doing
    6. Provide a resource list of support groups

V. **Spiritual Concerns**[2,6-7,16–21]

A. **Differences between religiosity and spirituality**
    1. Religion is a particular system of faith and worship
    2. Spirituality encompasses transcending the material and self to a higher power
        a) Feeling of interconnectedness with a higher power
        b) Meaning through a sense of relatedness to a higher power

B. **Holistic care: including spirituality provides holistic care through the body, mind, and spirit**

C. **Terminal illness creates an increased sense of vulnerability and mortality for everyone involved**

D. **Terminal illness also creates loss and suffering in various degrees**

E. **The need to find meaning in what is happening to the patient and to the caregiver**
    1. Meaning of dying
    2. Meaning of human existence
    3. Meaning of suffering
    4. Meaning of remaining days left

F. **Fear of the future of uncertainty and ambiguity**
    1. Life in general
    2. Own death
    3. Who will be their caregiver when the time comes
    4. Finances
    5. Love and security
    6. Loss of their role: "What will I be when I am no longer a caregiver?"

G. **Relatedness to God or whatever represents God**
    1. The concept of "God" or a superior being
    2. Comfort can come from the fact that "God" is more than human
    3. Need for rituals, sacraments, the exercising of beliefs

H. **Sense of hope**
    1. Linked to a sense of purpose
    2. Often directly proportional to the patient's status
    3. Related to a sense of connectedness to god or others
    4. Provides confidence in life after death, a sense of future
    5. Essential for day to day life, especially in these circumstances

I. **Interventions**
    1. Use active listening and presence
    2. Assess past spiritual support, religious practices, and resources
    3. Help construct a sense of hope
    4. Pray with and/or share scripture
    5. Provide, if desired, appropriate religious supports (e.g., priest, minister, rabbi)
    6. Provide help on the basis of individual needs

CITED REFERENCES

1. Duhamel F, Dupuis F. Guaranteed returns: investing in conversations with families of patients with cancer. *Clin J Oncol Nurs.* 2004;8(1):68–71.

2. Farber SJ, Egnew TR, Herman-Bertsch JL, Taylor TR, Guldin GE. Issues in end-of-life care: patient, caregiver, and clinician perceptions. *J Palliat Med.* 2003;6(1):19–31.

3. Ferrell BR. The family. In: Doyle D, Hanks G, MacDonald N, eds. *Oxford Textbook of Palliative Medicine.* Oxford, UK: Oxford Medical Publication; 2009:909–918.

4. Grunfeld E, Coyle D, Whelan T, et. al. Family caregiver burden: results of a longitudinal study of breast cancer patients and their principal caregivers. *Cmaj.* 2004;170(12):1795–1801.

5. Isaksen AS, Thuen F, Hanestad B. Patients with cancer and their close relatives: experiences with treatment, care, and support. *Cancer Nurs.* 2003;26(1):68–74.

6. Kemp C. *Terminal Illness: A Guide to Nursing Care.* Philadelphia, PA: J.B. Lippincott; 1999.

7. Borneman T. Caring for cancer patients at home: the effect on family caregivers. *Home Health Care Management & Practice.* 1998;10(4):25–33.

8. Hileman JW, Lackey NR. Self-identified needs of patients with cancer at home and their home caregivers: a descriptive study. *Oncol Nurs Forum.* 1990;17(6):907–913.

9. Steele RG, Fitch MI. Coping strategies of family caregivers of home hospice patients with cancer. *Oncol Nurs Forum.* 1996;23(6):955–960.

10. Steele RG, Fitch MI. Needs of family caregivers of patients receiving home hospice care for cancer. *Oncol Nurs Forum.* 1996;23(5):823–828.

11. Harding R, Higginson IJ. What is the best way to help caregivers in cancer and palliative care? A systematic literature review of interventions and their effectiveness. *Palliat Med.* 2003;17(1):63–74.

12. Vachon ML. Psychosocial needs of patients and families. *J Palliat Care.* 1998;14(3):49–56.

13. Abrahm JL. Update in palliative medicine and end-of-life care. *Annu Rev Med.* 2003;54:53–72.

14. Gorman L. The psychosocial impact of cancer on the individual, family, and society. In: Carroll-Johnson RM, Gorman L, Bush N, eds. *Psychosocial Nursing Care along the Cancer Continuum.* Pittsburgh, PA: Oncology Nursing Press, Inc.; 2006:3–23.

15. Ferszt B, Houck P. The family. In: Amenta MO, Bohnet NL, eds. *Nursing Care of the Terminally Ill.* Boston, MA: Little, Brown and Company; 1986:173–190.

16. Amenta MO. Spiritual concerns. In: Amenta MO, Bohnet NL, eds. *Nursing Care of the Terminally Ill.* Boston, MA: Little, Brown and Company; 1986:115–116.

17. Herth KA, Cutcliffe JR. The concept of hope in nursing 3: hope and palliative care nursing. *Br J Nurs.* 2002;11(14):977–983.

18. Speck P. Spiritual issues in palliative care. In: Doyle D, Hanks G, Macdonald N, eds. *Oxford Textbook of Palliative Medicine.* Oxford, UK: Oxford Medical Publication; 2009.

19. Taylor EJ. Spirituality and the cancer experience. In: Carroll-Johnson RM, Gorman L, Bush N, eds. *Psychosocial Nursing Care along the Cancer Continuum.* Pittsburgh, PA: Oncology Nursing Press, Inc.; 2006:117–131.

20. Taylor EJ. *Spiritual Care: Nursing Theory, Research, and Practice.* Upper Saddle River, NJ: Prentice-Hall; 2002.

21. Taylor EJ. Spiritual needs of patients with cancer and family caregivers. *Cancer Nurs.* 2003;26(4): 260–266.

ADDITIONAL REFERENCES AND RESOURCES

Borneman T, Stahl C, Ferrell B, Smith D. The concept of hope in family caregivers of cancer patients and home. *Journal of Hospice and Palliative Nursing.* 2002;4(1):21–33.

Clukey L. "Just be there": hospice caregivers' anticipatory mourning experience. *Journal of Hospice and Palliative Nursing.* 2007;9(3):150–158.

Coreless I. Bereavement. In: Ferrell BR, Coyle N, eds. *Textbook of Palliative Nursing.* 3rd ed. New York, NY: Oxford University Press; 2010:597–612.

Davis BA, Burns J, Rezac D, et al. Family stress and advance directives: a comparative study. *Journal of Hospice and Palliative Nursing.* 2005;7(4):219–227.

Family Caregiver Alliance. Available at: www.caregiver.org/caregiver/jsp/home.jsp.

Family Caregiver Support Network. Available at: www.caregiversupportnetwork.org/.

Johnson JO, Sulmasy DP, Nolan MT. Patients' experiences of being a burden on family in terminal illness. *Journal of Hospice and Palliative Nursing.* 2007;9(5):264–269.

Lowey SE. Communication between the nurse and family caregiver in end-of-life care: a review of the literature. *Journal of Hospice and Palliative Nursing.* 2008;10(1):35–45.

Kazanowski M. Family caregivers' medication management of symptoms in patients with cancer near death. *Journal of Hospice and Palliative Nursing.* 2005;7(3):174–181.

Kruse BG. The meaning of letting go: the lived experience for caregivers of persons at the end of life. *Journal of Hospice and Palliative Nursing.* 2004;6(4):215–222.

National Alliance for Caregiving. Available at: www.caregiving.org/.

National Family Caregivers Association. Available at: www.thefamilycaregiver.org/.

Wellisch DK, Kissane DW. Family issues and palliative care. In: Chochinov H, Breitbart W, eds. *Handbook of Psychiatry in Palliative Medicine.* 2nd ed. New York: Oxford University Press; 2009:220–235.

Chapter XI

Bereavement

Tami Borneman, RN, PHN, MSN, CNS, FPCN

I. Introduction: Definitions[1,2]

    A. Grief: intense, emotional loss caused by suffering; thoughts, feelings, and behaviors one experiences after a loss

    B. Mourning: the outward signs of grief; process one goes through adapting to a loss

    C. Bereavement: complex series of reactions following death, including grief and mourning; situation of losing to death a person or a loved one

    D. Attachment: a strong need to remain close to, or to return to, another individual

II. Stages/Process of Grief

    A. Bereavement Is a Process Unique to Each Individual

    B. The Nature of Grief[1]

        1. Urge to cry and to search for the deceased

        2. Avoiding or repressing crying or searching: social value of being taught to have a "stiff upper lip"

        3. Reviewing and revising internal models

           a) Death of a loved one can invalidate one's assumptions about the world, thought patterns, and behavior, which formerly included or depended on the deceased

           b) The familiar world becomes rather unfamiliar

           c) Often the process is initially resisted

C. **Anticipatory Grief**[3-6]

1. "Process of mourning, coping, interaction, planning, and psychosocial reorganization that is stimulated and begun in part in response to the awareness of the impending loss of a loved one and the recognition of associated losses in the past, present, and future"[5, p. 35]

2. Therapeutic aspects of anticipatory grieving involve balancing the equally conflicting emotions of simultaneously holding on, letting go, and drawing closer to their dying loved one

3. When the realization of death is reinforced by the illness progression and awareness gradually surfaces, one is said to have entered into the anticipatory phase[3]

4. Healthcare professionals at times experience anticipatory grieving. For example, the nurse may sense death is inevitable before the physician or family. The nurse begins anticipatory grieving while others are still focused on cure or prolonging life[3]

D. **Theoretical Tasks of Grief**

1. Kübler-Ross[7]

    a) Denial

    b) Anger

    c) Bargaining

    d) Depression

    e) Acceptance

2. Parkes[1]

    a) Alarm—physiological response

    b) Searching

    (1) Involves pangs of grief stimulated by memories of the loss

    (2) Bereaved may share having seen or heard or called out to the deceased

    c) Mitigation

    (1) Behaviors used to lessen the pain such as talking or praying to the deceased, denying the loss, increasing activity, returning to work

    (2) An attempt is made to make sense of the loss

    d) Anger and guilt

    (1) Anger usually occurs during the first year

    (2) Those with the greatest anger usually experience more isolation

    (3) Guilt over an aspect of the relationship can be a risk for complicated grief

    (4) Can arise from imagined omissions of duty, failure and negligence

    (5) May feel guilty of still being alive

    e) Gaining new identity: includes recovery of lost functions, adaptation to new roles and status and completion of acute grief

3. Bowlby[8]

    a) Numbing, with possible anguish and anger

    b) Searching and longing

    c) Disorganization and despair

    d) Reorganization

4. Wordon's Tasks[2]

    a) Accept reality of the loss

    b) Experience the pain of grief

    c) Adjust to an environment without the deceased

    d) Withdraw emotional energy and reinvest in another relationship

5. Rando's Process of Bereavement[5,6]

    a) Recognize the loss and death

    b) React to, experience and express the separation and pain

    c) Reminisce

    d) Relinquish old attachments

    e) Readjust and adapt to the new role while maintaining memories and form a new identity

    f) Reinvest

E. Demographics and Cultural Issues[1,3]

1. Be aware of cultural differences
2. Use guidelines and manuals to read about beliefs, customs and religions
3. Elicit information from the patient and family
4. Set aside own value judgments, avoid interjecting personal preference
5. Deaths of children and multiple deaths are regarded as the most severe types of loss
6. Women generally show emotions easier than men and are more inclined to seek help
7. Age

    a) Very young—difference between permanent and temporary separations is unclear

    b) Older children—similar to adults but can be complicated by failure in communication

    c) Old age—bereavement is less often unexpected, and because of the many losses encountered, it is sometimes considered to be a normal part of aging

III. Assessment[3]

A. Integrated into the conversation with the patient and family

B. Each answer to assessment questions (not merely probing) is a potential for teaching, therapeutic response, and intervention

C. Includes both verbal and nonverbal responses

D. Is coupled with nurturance, comfort, touch, gentle voice, impression one has unlimited time, and a sense of presence and compassion

IV. Interventions/Resources

A. Plan of Care[3,9,10]
1. Assessment
    a) Description of the death in the family's own words
    b) Concurrent stressors, past losses, reactions to their anniversaries
    c) Affective response (feelings, inability to concentrate)
    d) Somatic responses (sleep disturbances, poor appetite, pain, weakness, social withdrawal, hyperactivity)
    e) Support systems
    f) Financial concerns
    g) Past history of coping and psychiatric history
    h) Suicidal tendencies
    i) Alcohol or drug abuse: other substance abuse
    j) Spiritual/religious beliefs
    k) Cultural traditions
    l) Unusual experiences since death
2. Nursing Diagnoses[4,11]
    a) Bereavement
    b) Spiritual distress
    c) Dysfunctional grief
    d) Impaired adjustment
    e) Anxiety
    f) Ineffective individual coping
3. DSM-IV Diagnoses[12]
    a) Major depressive disorder
    b) Post-traumatic stress disorder

4. Expected outcomes
    a) Family will begin the grief process within own cultural norms and family traditions
    b) Family will share the grief reaction and its impact
    c) Family will seek support as needed
    d) In time, family will engage in life and other relationships

5. Interventions
    a) Provide continuous supportive listening and reassurance
    b) When appropriate, elicit a life review
    c) Provide privacy
    d) Encouragement of unfinished business and assist family in achieving desired goals
    e) Encourage use of cultural practices
    f) Offer spiritual support and referrals when needed
    g) Provide verbal and written information on the grief process and what to expect
    h) Use touch, holding and presence when appropriate
    i) Be sensitive for the need for silent presence
    j) Teach relaxation techniques
    k) Use guided imagery when appropriate
    l) Provide referrals for appropriate support groups as needed
    m) Encourage social support
    n) Encourage healthy coping mechanisms (e.g., exercise and rest)
    o) Give permission to grieve

B. **Complicated Grief**[1-3,5,6,13-15]

1. Those at risk for complicated grief
    a) Those who have an underlying low self-esteem
    b) Having had an ambivalent relationship
    c) Having had a dependent relationship (separation anxiety)
    d) Loss of role as caregiver especially if this role brought the patient and caregiver closer together
    e) Premature death
    f) Traumatic death
    g) Sudden death
    h) Death of an organ or bone marrow transplant recipient
    i) Death by suicide or homicide
    j) Death of a child
    k) Financial loss as a result of the terminal illness

2. Examples of complicated grief
    a) Prolonged/chronic grief: memories/conversations stir up uncontrollable weeping even years after the death
    b) Absent grief: no show of grief and sadness
    c) Exaggerated grief: self-destructive behaviors such as suicide
    d) Masked grief: bereaved is unaware of the behaviors that interfere with normal functioning
    e) Depression
    f) Post-traumatic stress disorder
3. Complicated grief can cause problems in relationships with family/friends

C. **Unusual Experiences**[3]
1. Bereaved having felt they have had contact with the deceased family member
    a) Often discounted as dreams or hallucinations
    b) Often judged as being "out there"
    c) Actual incidence is not known, but suspected to be more frequent than is shared
    d) Mourners may feel they are going crazy because they see or hear things others do not
    e) May create a fear of losing reality
2. Therapeutic effects
    a) Affirmation of the death
    b) Completion of unfinished business
    c) Sense that their loved one is alright
    d) Reduction in their own suffering
3. Interventions
    a) Encouraging sharing of unusual events, both for colleagues and family members
    b) Do not pass judgment
    c) Do not dismiss or label as hallucinations

V. Recognition of Staff Grief

A. **Nature of the Patient/Nurse Relationship**[3,15,16]
1. The loss is mourned regardless of the type of relationship experienced (e.g., close, ambivalent or hostile)
2. Nurses may become callous, but are not immune to grief

3. Sometimes grief over a close patient relationship results in a culmination of grief experienced from many deaths

B. Coping

1. Good deaths

    a) Nurses cope better with what they consider to have been a good death

    b) Death considered good if

        (1) Symptoms were managed

        (2) It was felt that the best possible care was given

        (3) Patient came to some resolution

        (4) Death did not violate a natural order (e.g., not a child or young adult)

2. Deaths considered bad if

    a) Nurse/family members were not present at time of death

    b) Grief characterized as painful, complicated, distressing or difficult

3. Anger

    a) Not an uncommon response to continual exposure to death

    b) Poorly tolerated in our culture

    c) Increased if one feels responsible for not curing, eliminating symptoms or for *causing* side effects from symptom management

    d) Acknowledging anger can help the nurse deal with feelings of depression and guilt

C. Self-Care[3,16,17]

1. Most important is initiating action on individual, managerial and institutional levels to help staff cope with grief

2. Specific interventions

    a) Support groups

    b) Self-assessment of numbers of deaths and toll taken

    c) Assessment of other areas of stress

    d) Acknowledge limitations and set appropriate boundaries

    e) Do not be afraid to ask for help

    f) Assess participation in positive aspects of one's life such as spirituality, play, sexuality, laughter, hobbies

    g) Provide/create ceremonies and programs that serve to acknowledge grief for both professionals and families

    h) Send bereavement cards or call the family

VI. Conclusion

A. Bereavement does not begin after death, but rather in events leading up to the death

B. Nurses have wonderful opportunities to care for the bereaved through listening, assisting in communications, teaching families about the process of dying or facilitating bereavement support groups

C. Bereavement provides nurses with opportunities to prevent ill health and to help families find new directions for growth

D. Grief is changing and dynamic

E. Grief is experienced physiologically, psychologically, socially, and spiritually

F. Spiritually, families have a need to be comforted by those sharing the same faith, have a need for prayer, and to feel supported by God and others

CITED REFERENCES

1. Parks C. Bereavement. In: Doyle D, Hanks G, MacDonald N, eds. *Oxford Textbook of Palliative Medicine*. 2nd ed. Oxford, UK: Oxford Medical Publication; 2009:995–1012.

2. El-Jawahri AR, Prigerson HG. Bereavement care. In: Berger A, Portenoy R, Weissman D, eds. *Principles & Practice of Palliative Care & Supportive Oncology*. 3rd ed. Philadelphia, PA: Lippincott Williams & Wilkins; 2007:645–653.

3. Brown-Saltzman K. Transforming the grief experience. In: Carroll-Johnson RM, Gorman L, Bush N, eds. *Psychosocial Nursing Care along the Cancer Continuum*. Pittsburgh, PA: Oncology Nursing Press, Inc.; 2006:293–314.

4. Duke S. An exploration of anticipatory grief: the lived experience of people during their spouses' terminal illness and in bereavement. *J Adv Nurs*. 1998;28(4):829–839.

5. Rando T. *Treatment of Complicated Mourning*. Champaign, IL: Research Press; 1993.

6. Rando T. *Clinical Dimensions of Anticipatory Mourning*. Champaign, IL: Research Press; 2000.

7. Kübler-Ross E. *On Death and Dying*. New York, NY: Macmillan; 1969.

8. Bowlby J. *Attachment and Loss*. New York, NY: Basic Books; 1980.

9. Foley G. *Lessons from the Bereaved: Care for the Dying*. Paper presented at the Sixth National Conference on Cancer Nursing, Seattle, WA; 1991.

10. Forte AL, Hill M, Pazder R, Feudtner C. Bereavement care interventions: a systematic review. *BMC Palliat Care*. 2004;3(1):3.

11. North American Nursing Diagnosis Association. *Nursing Diagnoses: Definitions and Classification*. Philadelphia, PA: North American Nursing Diagnosis Association; 2007–2008.

12. American Psychiatric Association. *Diagnostic and Statistical Manual of Mental Disorders*. 4th ed. Washington, DC: American Psychiatric Association; 2000.

13. Bohnet N. Bereavement care. In: Amenta M, Bohnet N, eds. *Nursing Care of the Terminally Ill*. Boston, MA: Little, Brown and Company; 1986.

14. Kemp C. *Terminal Illness: A Guide to Nursing Care*. Philadelphia, PA: J.B. Lippincott Company; 1999.

15. Loney M. Death, dying, and grief in the face of cancer. In: Burke C, ed. *Psychosocial Dimensions of Oncology Nursing Care*. Pittsburgh, PA: Oncology Nursing Press, Inc.; 1998:152–179.

16. Vachon M, Sherwood C. Staff stress and burnout. In: Berger A, Portenoy R, Weissman D, eds. *Principles & Practice of Palliative Care & Supportive Oncology*. 2nd ed. Philadelphia, PA: Lippincott Williams & Wilkins; 2007:667–686.

17. Lo K, Causey B, Crandall F. *Care at the Time of Death*. Paper presented at the Hospice Training Program, Largo, FL; 1996.

Additional References and Resources

Ailey SH, O'Rourke M, Breakwell S, Murphy A. Supporting a community of individuals with intellectual and developmental disabilities in grieving. *Journal of Hospice and Palliative Nursing.* 2008;10(5):285–292.

Bloch S, Kissane DW. Family-focused grief therapy. In: Chochinov H, Breitbart W, eds. *Handbook of Psychiatry in Palliative Medicine.* 2nd ed. New York, NY: Oxford University Press; 2009:504–518.

Brady EM. Unspeakable: the truth about grief. *Journal of Hospice and Palliative Nursing.* 2005;7(1):13–14.

Coreless I. Bereavement. In: Ferrell BR, Coyle N, eds. *Textbook of Palliative Nursing.* 3rd ed. New York, NY: Oxford University Press; 2010:597–612.

Eaves YD, McQuiston C, Miles MS. Coming to terms with adult sibling grief: when a brother dies from aids. *Journal of Hospice and Palliative Nursing.* 2005;7(3):139–149.

Glazer HR, Clark MD, Stein DS. The impact of hippotherapy on grieving children. *Journal of Hospice and Palliative Nursing.* 2004;6(3):171–175.

Kehl KA. Recognition and support of anticipatory mourning. *Journal of Hospice and Palliative Nursing.* 2005;7(4):206–211.

Neimeyer RA, Pennebaker JW, van Dyke JG. Narrative medicine: writing through bereavement. In: Chochinov H, Breitbart W, eds. *Handbook of Psychiatry in Palliative Medicine.* 2nd ed. New York, NY: Oxford University Press; 2009:454–469.

Romesberg TL. Understanding grief: a component of neonatal palliative care. *Journal of Hospice and Palliative Nursing.* 2002;6(3):161–170.

Scannell-Desch E. Prebereavement and postbereavement struggles and triumphs of midlife widows. *Journal of Hospice and Palliative Nursing.* 2002;7(1):15–22.

Steeves RH, Kahn DL. Experiences of bereavement in rural elders. *Journal of Hospice and Palliative Nursing.* 2005;7(4):197–205.

Thornburg P, Schim SM, Paige V, Grubaugh K. Nurses' experiences of caring while letting go. *Journal of Hospice and Palliative Nursing.* 2008;10(6):382–391.

Wright PM, Hogan NS. Grief theories and models: applications to hospice nursing practice. *Journal of Hospice and Palliative Nursing.* 2008;10(6):350–356.

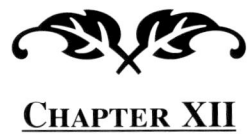

CHAPTER XII

CARE AT THE TIME OF DYING

Jeanne Martinez, RN, MPH, CHPN®, FPCN
Marianne Matzo, PhD, GNP-BC, FPCN, FAAN

Adapted from: Martinez J, Matzo ML. Care of the patient and family when death is nearing. In: Ersek M, ed. *Core Curriculum for the Hospice and Palliative Nursing Assistant*, Dubuque, IA: Kendall Hunt Publishing; 2003:59–69.

I. Introduction/Overview

    A. Once it is determined that a patient is dying and treatment to cure the disease is no longer helpful, providing comfort care ensures a peaceful death

    B. Nursing can do much to make this time comfortable; there is only one chance for us to do this well for each person

    C. Care should be individualized to each patient's needs and goals, as much as possible

    D. Even very ill patients can be given control over their immediate surroundings

    E. Patients need ongoing monitoring of their symptoms; ask if the patient is satisfied with how well their symptoms are controlled

    F. Providing excellent care at the time of dying includes emotional support of family members and consists of listening and being present for people as they grieve the loss of their loved one

    G. The major ways to ensure good care to dying patients and to support their families is by

        1. Making the environment as comfortable as possible

        2. Giving care with an attitude of attentiveness, compassion and concern to the individual patient and the family

        3. Working with the team to avoid any burdensome care, such as unnecessary weights, taking vital signs or other care that may cause discomfort to the patient

4. Respecting patient's and family's cultural, religious, and other values without judging them or imposing personal beliefs

5. Working as a team member by sharing observations, reporting problems and concerns, and supporting each other

H. When done well, care of the dying can be very rewarding

II. Patient and Family Needs and Goals Related to the Dying Process

A. Assist the patient to meet his or her end-of-life goals; ask patient the following questions

1. Who does the patient want to be there?

2. What are the most important needs and goals for the patient before death?

    a) Prioritize care according to the patient's (then the family's) goals

    b) If there is conflict in what patients and family members want, patient desires come first

3. Where does the patient want to die?

4. Inform other team members about the patient's and family's wishes and goals; it may take the entire team to work together to meet patient's goals, for example, to arrange discharge and hospice services if the patient wants to die at home instead of in the hospital

B. Cultural influences (see Chapters VII and VIII)

1. Determine important beliefs and values that affect patient's goals

2. Respect the need for a patient to die on his or her own terms

3. Never impose your own religious or cultural beliefs on a patient or family

4. Avoid judging how family members cope with loss and death, and express their grief

C. Family needs

1. Who is the patient's family or support system?

2. Do patient and family goals conflict?

3. Report conflicting goals and values to the team

4. Assist patients and family members to "reframe hope," for example, help family and patients to meet short-term goals focused on hopes at end of life, such as the hope to have a pain-free day, or the hope of seeing a new grandchild born

D. Re-evaluation

1. Periodically reassess patient goals; help patients to decide what is most important to them

2. Continually check patients for unresolved symptoms

3. Frequently monitor the effectiveness of medications and other interventions and whether patients are satisfied with symptom management

4. Always share patient's and family's wishes, concerns and need for further intervention with the team

III. The Environment[1]

A. Immediate Physical Environment

1. Respect the environment as a sacred space; that is, as a place where a profound change is to occur

2. Individualize the environment; determine what is important and meaningful to the patient or family related to the following

   a) Objects and views

   (1) What objects are meaningful (for example, photos, rosary beads, books, pillows)?

   (2) What should be in the patient's line of vision should he or she awaken?

   (3) What about window views?

   (4) Can the bed be repositioned to improve the patient's environment?

   (5) If the patient is at home, is he or she isolated in a bedroom (and is that what they want) or is he or she in a central room of the home (and is that what they want)?

   b) Lighting

   (1) Is natural light available?

   (2) Is room lighting harsh or gentle?

   c) Sound

   (1) Is the room too noisy?

   (2) Does the patient respond differently to various noise levels?

   (3) Provide music, TV, other sounds that the patient likes, as the patient desires

   (4) Vary the noise environment to enhance the patient's comfort and promote natural sleep cycles

   (5) Provide or increase calming sounds. Decrease or stop sounds that disturb the patient

   d) Family space in a facility

   (1) Can the environment be made less sterile or medical? Is it welcoming to families and visitors?

   (2) Are there comfortable chairs for family members and other visitors?

   (3) Is there a close common space for family members when they are not in the patient's room?

   (4) Are coffee, water or other refreshments available nearby?

(5) Is a phone or cell phone area available nearby, but outside of the patient's room, for family use?

(6) Does the environment promote privacy as much as possible?

B. **Staff Behaviors and Attitudes**

1. Frequently visit the dying patient's room

2. Maintain a balance between giving family members privacy and being there for support

3. Sit down when talking with the patient or family members

4. Listen carefully to the patient's and family members' issues; express your compassion and concern

5. Stress may prevent family members from listening or remembering what you tell them; they may need the same questions answered many times. Communicate with the healthcare team to ensure that the patient and family are given consistent answers and explanations

6. Recognize the importance of your presence, that is, being versus doing; role-model this behavior for families and other staff

IV. **Symptom Management Related to Decline in Status**

A. **Goals of care: watch for new or note existing symptoms or problems; ask the patient which problems cause the most concern**

B. **Common symptoms in patients near the time of death (also see Chapters IV and V)**

1. Agitation/restlessness

   a) The person may make restless and repetitive motions, such as pulling at bed linen or clothing

   b) Observe for reversible physical causes, such as full bladder, constipation, impaction

   c) Consider that the cause of restlessness or distress may be emotional or spiritual in nature

   d) Nursing actions

   (1) Speak in a quiet, natural way

   (2) Lightly massage the patient's forehead, back, or arms, if acceptable to patient

   (3) Read to the person

   (4) Play some soothing music

   (5) Try to decrease the number of people around the bedside, if this increases the patient's agitation

   (6) Avoid asking a lot of questions or talking a lot

   (7) Do not interfere with or try to restrain restless motions, unless the patient is harming himself or herself

   (8) Provide sedative and pain medications as ordered

2. Pain

   a) Observe for moaning, restlessness, furrowing of the brow and grimacing, which may indicate pain or discomfort

   b) Continue or begin non-drug pain therapies such as

      (1) Gentle massage

      (2) Repositioning the patient

      (3) Pleasant diversions, such as music, being read to, etc.

      (4) For some patients, company and distraction can help pain, but for others a calm, quiet environment works better; observe patients for what seems to provide the most comfort. Communicate this to the healthcare team

      (5) Provide pain medications as ordered, with continued assessment for effectiveness. As the body is shutting down, and unable to clear medications, it may be necessary to decrease medication doses, and change from long-acting to short-acting opioids[1]

3. Dyspnea

   a) Difficulty breathing, feeling short of breath

      (1) Cheyne-Stokes breathing pattern is characterized by uneven shallow breathing alternating with periods of apnea. It is a common respiratory pattern prior to death[2]

   b) Can be very distressing to patients and families

   c) Nursing actions

      (1) Positioning: put the head of the bed up; put pillows behind the patient's head; and if possible, sit the patient up in a reclining chair

      (2) Suggest that the patient move more slowly; keep still, lay quietly; and use pursed-lip or deep, slower breathing

      (3) Direct a fan to the face or open a window (or both) to move air through the patient's room

      (4) Use relaxation or distraction techniques with the patient

      (5) Short-acting morphine or other opioids help to decrease the feelings of breathlessness[2]

      (6) Oxygen therapy does not usually relieve dyspnea at the end of life, though it may be useful if the patient feels it is[2]

4. Noisy respirations or "death rattle"

   a) Caused by relaxation of throat muscles and pooling of secretions

   b) More disturbing to families than patient

   c) Nursing actions

      (1) Frequently change patient's position

(2) Provide support to the families; assure them that noisy breathing does not mean the patient is in distress; avoid using the term "death rattle" with or in the presence of the patient and/or family

(3) Use medications to calm breathing or decrease secretions as ordered

5. Anorexia and dysphagia

   a) Anorexia: lack of appetite

   b) Dysphagia: difficulty swallowing

   c) Result of the process of the body "shutting down"

      (1) Can cause the family distress; conflict can occur because the issues of nutrition and hydration are very emotional for family members

   d) Nursing actions

      (1) Offer conscious patients small frequent sips of fluids or bits of soft food followed by mouth care

         i. If having difficulty swallowing, a consultation with a nutritionist or speech therapist may be helpful depending on the patient's status and ability to participate

      (2) For unconscious patients, provide frequent, gentle mouth care

      (3) Help families to cope with the changes in patient status. Reinforce that the goals of eating are for patient comfort and pleasure, as weight gain and weight maintenance are usually not achievable at end stage. In addition, artificial hydration and feeding can cause distressing symptoms, such as edema, fluid overload, nausea, vomiting, and diarrhea

C. General comfort care for patients nearing death[3]

1. Oral care

   a) Keep the patient's mouth moist

      (1) Rinse the patient's mouth frequently with water

      (2) Keep room humidified using spray bottle or humidifier

      (3) Use commercially available salivary substitutes or supplements (e.g., Salivart®, Salagen®, MoiStir®)

   b) Apply lip lubricant or mineral oil generously to patient's lips

   c) Keep patient's mouth and teeth clean

      (1) Use soft-bristled toothbrushes or sponge-covered oral swabs with non-abrasive toothpaste to brush teeth

      (2) Tongue blade wrapped in gauze and moistened may be used as an alternative to a toothbrush

      (3) Keep dentures and bridges clean; do not insert if patient has mouth sores

(4) Avoid alcohol-based mouthwashes and lemon glycerin swabs because of drying and unpleasant taste

(5) Frequently rinse mouth; mouth rinses using, for example, baking soda in water or saline rinses, chlorhexidine 0.2% (Peridex®)

(6) If the patient is able to swallow, provide small chips of ice, frozen Gatorade™, or juice in small amounts by spoon or syringe, to refresh the patient

(7) Carefully monitor for changes in the ability to swallow. Ensure that all family and healthcare team members are aware if a patient should NOT receive oral intake due to dysphagia to avoid aspiration

d) Use topical (applied to the skin and mucous membranes) anesthetics (medications that numb an area, for example, lidocaine) for mouth sores

2. Elimination management

a) Use absorbent pads/adult diapers

b) Apply moisture barrier to the skin

c) Indwelling catheter for large amounts of urinary incontinence

d) For fecal incontinence, assess for underlying causes, such as impaction, laxatives and tube feedings

3. Skin integrity

a) Watch for skin breakdown, especially in bony areas, such as shoulder blades, elbows, heels, back of head, over the ears and lower spine

b) Prevent skin breakdown and discomfort through properly positioning the patient in bed and frequently turning the patient

c) Be aware of the possible need to medicate the patient prior to turning her or him

d) Anticipate the need for a special pressure mattress for comfort and skin breakdown prevention before a patient declines; this action may reduce the need for turning the patient as frequently in the final days or hours of life

e) Use a turning sheet for lifting and turning the patient

f) If patient has skin breakdown

(1) Prevent further breakdown by carefully positioning the patient and frequently changing the patient's position

(2) Observe the patient for pain or discomfort from the skin breakdown

(3) Keep the area of the breakdown clean

(4) Apply dressings as ordered

(5) Control wound odors by gently cleansing the area, applying and changing dressings appropriately, keeping room well ventilated, and using room deodorizers if necessary

V. Psychosocial and Spiritual Issues

A. Psychosocial Support for the Patient

1. Allow patients as much control over their environment and caregiving as possible
2. Maintain patient dignity
    a) Assume that the patient can hear all conversations; speak directly to the patient, even if she or he does not respond
    b) Adjust language; for example, speaking of "diapers" is not dignified
    c) Avoid speaking to others as if the patient were not present
3. Be aware of possible fears commonly experienced at the end of life, for example, fear of
    a) The unknown
    b) Being abandoned
    c) Being a burden to one's family or support system
4. Communication/support
    a) Listen carefully and address the patient's concerns
    b) Orient the patient frequently, even if patient is non-communicative
    c) Periodically assess the non-verbal patient's ability to communicate by other means, such as squeezing hands or blinking

B. Psychosocial Support for the Family

1. Listen carefully and address family concerns
2. Allow the family as much control over the environment as possible
3. When multiple family members are involved, be aware of who has the role of decision-maker; and consult with that person regarding changes and decisions about the patient
4. Some families want to be present throughout the period when the patient is dying, whereas others are uncomfortable being near the person; respect individual preferences[1]
5. Common family fears at time of the death of a loved one[2]
    a) Being alone with the patient
    b) Having to watch patient suffer, or experience a painful death
    c) Being alone with patient when death occurs, and fear of their own responses
    d) Not knowing when the patient has died
    e) Causing the patient's death by giving medications (in home care setting)

C. Grieving (also see Chapter XI)

1. Grief
    a) Is an individual, emotional response to a loss

b) Is a process that is not orderly or predictable

c) Begins before the death occurs and continues after the death of the patient

2. The grieving person never "gets over" a loss, but can heal and learn to live with a loss and live without the deceased

3. Nursing actions

   a) Education and preparation

      (1) Keep the family informed of the patient's status, the care you have provided, and any interactions with the patient

      (2) Reinforce information the family has received for what to expect as the patient becomes closer to death

      (3) Provide information on grieving to help normalize the process

      (4) Inform other healthcare team members of the patient's or family's questions and concerns

   b) Caregiving

      (1) If the family desires, encourage them to participate in caregiving

      (2) If family does not want to provide care or is emotionally or physically tired, give them permission to take a break and allow others to provide patient care

      (3) By providing good care at the end of life, you help the patient to have a good death, which also eases later grieving for the family

   c) Grief coaching and resources

      (1) Encourage families to communicate with the patient before death, even if the patient cannot respond

      (2) Suggest that family members may wish to say good-bye when leaving the person, as death is unpredictable

      (3) Provide resources for available bereavement support

      (4) Provide spiritual support and referrals to clergy, as appropriate

      (5) Respect the patient and family members' spiritual and cultural beliefs and values. Never impose your own beliefs on others

D. **Other Issues around Dying**[4]

   1. Requests or plans to end a person's life through euthanasia or assisted suicide. With an actively dying person, this request is most likely to come from a distressed family member, than the patient. In either case, you need to be prepared to do the following

      a) Respond to the request in a non-judgmental, calm, and supportive way

      b) Never make a promise to keep such requests or knowledge of a plan from other members of the patient's healthcare team

      c) Report such requests, conversations, or plans <u>immediately</u> to your supervisor or the person in charge

d) Know your agency's policy for responding to such a request. Euthanasia and Physician Assisted Suicide (PAS) are illegal in the United States, except in the states of Oregon and Washington. Those states have specific protocols for how to process such a request

e) Participate with the healthcare team's plan on any changes in the care plan needed to best help the suffering of the patient and family, which caused this request[5]

2. The "final rally"

   a) Days or hours before death, a non-verbal or comatose patient may suddenly awaken for a short time, be able to speak or even eat a meal

   b) This behavior is usually temporary, but may confuse family members into thinking the patient is "doing better"

3. Symbolic language

   a) Patient may talk about "preparing to go home," "going on a trip," or "standing in line"

   b) Although the patient may seem confused, some healthcare professionals see this as a normal process for some, referred to as "near-death awareness"

4. Vision-like experiences

   a) A person may experience seeing or speaking to someone who has already died; he or she may also see places not presently visible to others

   b) This normal process may reflect that the person is detaching from this life and is preparing for death

   c) Do not contradict, explain, belittle or argue about what the person claims to see or hear

5. Inability of the patient to "let go" and allow death to occur. At times, the family or healthcare professionals may wonder why the dying process of a very end stage person is so prolonged

   a) This may indicate that something emotional or spiritual for the patient is still unresolved or unfinished

   b) Report your observations to the team, to provide the best resources to identify what may be happening, and help the patient in the best way

6. Saying good-bye

   a) When the person is ready to die and the family is able to do so, saying good-bye is a final gift of love

   b) Saying good-bye helps family and friends in their grieving process

   c) It may be helpful to encourage the family to hold or touch the patient and say the things that they want to say

      (1) The message may be as simple (or as complicated) as saying, "I love you"

      (2) May include recounting favorite memories, places, and activities that were shared

(3) May include saying "I'm sorry for whatever I've done to cause any tensions or difficulty"

(4) Family members may also want to say "Thank you" and "I will miss you"

(5) Tears and crying are normal and natural parts of saying good-bye, and expressing loss and sadness; assure grieving people that there is no need to apologize or try to hide tears and sadness

7. Dying alone

   a) Family members may have a goal of being at the patient's bedside at the time of death and are upset it they are not present when the patient dies

   b) If this happens, gently explain this is not an uncommon occurrence

VI. Death

A. Signs that death is very near (hours or days) include

1. Changes in mentation

   a) Psychological and physical withdrawal

   b) Increased periods of sleeping

   c) Decreased consciousness, with difficulty or inability to awaken

2. Lack of eyelash reflex indicates deep coma

3. Decreased and concentrated (dark) urinary output resulting from decreased blood circulation to the kidneys

4. Skin coolness; hands, arms, feet, and legs become increasingly cool

5. Changes in skin color; paleness and sometimes presence of a bluish color resulting from decreased blood circulation, also called mottling

6. Incontinence; control of urine or bowels (or both) may be lost as the muscles in those areas begin to relax

7. Breathing pattern changes

   a) The person's regular breathing pattern may change and become irregular (e.g., shallow breaths with periods of no breathing for 5 to 30 seconds, up to a full minute, known as Cheyne-Stokes breathing)

   b) Noisy respirations, death rattle

   c) Apnea, which is a period of no breathing

   d) Reinforce to family members that the above breathing patterns are an expected part of the dying process, and usually not distressful to patients

B. How will you know when death has occurred?

1. The signs of death include such things as

   a) No heartbeat

   b) Bowel and bladder incontinence

      c) No response

      d) Eyelids slightly open

      e) Pupils enlarged, do not respond to changes in light

      f) Eyes fixed on a certain spot

      g) No blinking

      h) Jaw relaxed and mouth slightly open

2. Talk with the family about what they should do if they are alone with the patient when the death occurs

      a) The death of a hospice patient is expected and does not require an "emergency intervention." However, it often does require intense support for family at the bedside

      b) Family or you should notify the team (hospice, on-call or unit)

      c) A nurse or physician will verify the absence of vital signs, and/or pronounce the death. Then family members not present need to be notified, as well as the primary healthcare provider and the funeral home

      d) If possible the body should not be removed until the family is ready to leave it

3. Realize that even if the dying process is prolonged, you and the family may still feel "shocked" that the person has died when they did

4. Aftercare rituals and family support

      a) Position the body in an appropriate way for family viewing

      b) Help, as needed, with any cultural or religious rituals that the family desires

      c) Encourage family to spend time with the body, saying good-byes

      d) Ask if other family, friends, or clergy needs to come to view the body before it is removed from the room

      e) Reinforce information given to the family about what to expect immediately after death

          (1) Rigor mortis (stiffening of the body after death) occurs 2 to 4 hours after death, which may include the following

              i. Air may escape lungs, especially when turning the body; assure family that this does not mean the patient is still alive

              ii. Bowel and bladder incontinence commonly occur following death

5. Post-mortem care: care of the body after death

      a) Handle the body with the same respect you would if the person were alive

      b) Clean and groom the body as appropriate

      c) Ask if the family would like to participate in post-mortem care; some family members find it comforting to perform this last act of care for a loved one; in some cultures and for some relationships (such as the death of a child), family participation in preparation of the body may be very important

        d) Giving post-mortem care provides a good opportunity for you to say your own "good-byes" to the patient

        e) Prepare family members for the removal of the body from the room or home; this is often a difficult process to observe and families may wish to say good-byes and leave the area prior to the body being removed

VII. Professional Caregiver Coping with Care of the Dying

    A. Recognize the importance of professional coping and self-care when working with the dying

    B. Reframe your view of dying, so that death is an expected part of your practice

    C. Acknowledge and explore your personal feelings about patients who die; find what works best for your own coping with dying and grieving

    D. Recognize your limits and ask for help when you need it

    E. Assist others on the healthcare team who seem to be struggling emotionally with patient deaths or other issues

VIII. Conclusion

    A. Assist the patient to meet his or her own end-of-life goals (who, what, where)

    B. Enhance and individualize the environment

    C. Anticipate and monitor symptom management related to decline in status

    D. Anticipate the psychosocial and spiritual care needs of patients and families

    E. Aid family grieving

    F. Recognize the importance of professional coping and self-care in working with the dying

CITED REFERENCES

1. American Association of Colleges of Nursing and the City of Hope National Medical Center. Module 8: Preparation and care for the time of death. *End-of-Life Nursing Education Consortium (ELNEC) Project.* 2009. Funded through the Robert Wood Johnson Foundation.

2. Matzo M, Hill JA. Peri-death nursing care. In: Matzo ML, Sherman DW, eds. *Palliative Care Nursing: Quality Care to the End of Life.* New York, NY: Springer Publishing Company; 2010: 541–561.

3. De Conno F, Shanotto A, Ripamonte C, Ventafridda V. Mouth care. In: Doyle D, Hanks G, Cherny NI, Calman K, eds. *Oxford Textbook of Palliative Medicine.* 3rd ed. New York, NY: Oxford University Press; 2005:673–687.

4. Callahan M, Kelley P. *Final Gifts: Understanding the Special Awareness, Needs, & Communications of the Dying.* New York, NY: Bantam Books; 1992.

5. Stanley KJ, Zoloth-Dorfman L. Ethical considerations. In: Ferrell BR, Coyle N, eds. *Textbook of Palliative Nursing.* 2nd ed. New York, NY: Oxford University Press; 2006:1031–1053.

ADDITIONAL REFERENCES AND RESOURCES

Boucher J, Bova C, Sullivan-Bolyai S, et al. Next-of-kin's perspectives of end-of-life care. *Journal of Hospice and Palliative Nursing.* 2010;12(1):41–50.

Forbes MA, Rosdahl DR. The final journey of life. *Journal of Hospice and Palliative Nursing.* 2002;5(4):213–220.

Gauthier D. The meaning of healing near the end of life. *Journal of Hospice and Palliative Nursing.* 2002;4(4):220–227.

Halliday LE, Boughton MA. The moderating effect of death experience on death anxiety: implications for nursing education. *Journal of Hospice and Palliative Nursing.* 2008;10(2):76–82.

Kruse BG. The meaning of letting go: the lived experience for caregivers of persons at the end of life. *Journal of Hospice and Palliative Nursing.* 2002;6(4):215–222.

Ternestedt BM, Andershed B, Eriksson M, Johansson I. A good death: development of a nursing model of care. *Journal of Hospice and Palliative Nursing.* 2002;4(3):153–160.

Woods AB. The terror of the night: posttraumatic stress disorder at the end of life. *Journal of Hospice and Palliative Nursing.* 2002;5(4):196–204.

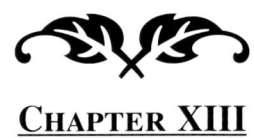

Chapter XIII

Personal and Professional Development

Dena Jean Sutermaster, RN, MSN, CHPN®
Judy Lentz, RN, MSN, NHA

Adapted from: Poleto MA. Personal and professional development. In: Ersek M, ed. *Core Curriculum for the Hospice and Palliative Nursing Assistant*. Dubuque, IA: Kendall Hunt Publishing; 2003:115–123.
and
Rooney EC, Poleto M. Interdisciplinary collaborative practice in the hospice and palliative care setting. In: Volker BG, Watson AC. eds. *Core Curriculum for the Generalist Hospice and Palliative Nurse*. Dubuque, IA: Kendall Hunt Publishing; 2002:15–28.

I. Introduction[1]

    A. Advances in the care of patients and family are always being developed

    B. Licensed practical/vocational nurses must meet the basic education and training requirements for the licensed practical/vocational nurse job and also to remain current with information and procedures that are specific to the needs of the seriously ill and dying

    C. Professional responsibilities go beyond maintaining one's competency and include other roles, such as advocating for patients, families, and colleagues; mentoring other licensed practical/vocational nurses and nursing assistants; and participating in activities aimed at improving care for seriously ill and dying patients and their families

II. Definitions

    A. Professionalism[2]

        1. As defined by National Board of Medical Examiners, professionalism is represented by the following characteristics

            a) Altruism

            b) Integrity

            c) Caring/compassion/communication

            d) Respect

e) Responsibility/accountability

f) Excellence/scholarship

g) Leadership

2. Using this model for nurses practicing in end-of-life care, the professional nurse should demonstrate the following behaviors

a) Altruism: put the patient/family first, continually advocate for the patient/family, be a team player promoting successful outcomes, participate in community activities that address end-of-life issues, and participate in local/national professional organizations

b) Integrity: be truthful, do not withhold information, balance humility with authority, maintain professional autonomy

c) Caring/compassion/communication: know when to listen, when to talk and when to seek additional information, break bad news with compassion; demonstrate compassion in every situation, show empathy

d) Respect: respect patient/family rights requesting permission with any invasion of privacy, respect differences in culture, tradition, backgrounds, etc., maintain personal boundaries

e) Responsibility/accountability: demonstrate reliability and accountability for responsibilities, be compliant with regulations and policies, be accountable for shortcomings, accept and provide constructive feedback, demonstrate ethical behaviors, control emotions with adversity

f) Excellence/scholarship: be committed, conscientious, thorough, use good decision-making skills, and continually seek to improve oneself scholastically

g) Leadership: lead and mentor others, actively participate in activities within the specialty locally and nationally when possible, advocate for the profession, seek to grow professionally in every aspect, commit to the code of conduct, demonstrate competence and follow the standards of care and professional behavior as written for the specialty

B. Scope of Practice[1,3]

1. Activities the licensed practice/vocational nurse is legally permitted to perform as determined by their state board of nursing

2. Scope of hospice and palliative care licensed practical/vocational nurse is the distinct body of knowledge that directs the licensed practical/vocational nurse in providing hospice and palliative care

3. It is imperative that licensed practical/vocational nurses who work in hospice and palliative care accept professional practice accountability and make certain that their practice remain within the scope of professional practice standards

4. Licensed practical/vocational nurses practicing palliative care must have multidimensional skills and practice under the direction of a registered nurse

5. Licensed practical/vocational nurses can take on a variety of roles based on the needs of their patients and families

C. **Hospice and Palliative Standards of Care**[3]

1. Identifies the responsibilities for which the hospice and palliative care licensed practical/vocational nurse is accountable

2. Describe a competent level of licensed practical/vocational nursing care as demonstrated by the nursing process

D. *Competencies for the Hospice and Palliative Care Licensed Practical/Vocational Nurse*[4]

1. In the *Competencies for the Hospice and Palliative Licensed Practical/Vocational Nurse*, a professional is defined as one who "demonstrates knowledge, attitudes, behaviors, and skills that are consistent with the scope of practice for hospice and palliative licensed practical/vocational nursing."[4, p. 3] The core competencies for professionalism in hospice and palliative nursing as defined by the Hospice and Palliative Nurses Association are

    a) Recognizes that influence of personal spiritual and cultural values on perceptions regarding dying and death and their impact on the quality of hospice and palliative care

    b) Demonstrates caring behavior and interpersonal connectiveness while maintaining personal and professional boundaries

    c) Demonstrates professional accountability to patients, families, colleagues, and institutions

    d) Engages in nursing activities that are appropriate to personal education, experience, and scope of practice

    e) Supports the advancement of hospice/palliative nursing through membership in HPNA and other professional organizations and participation in hospice and palliative education and community activities

    f) Participates in ongoing educational activities and certification to promote professional development

    g) Seeks constructive feedback regarding one's own professional practice through participation on performance evaluation, peer review and interactions with colleagues

    h) Maintains physical, social, emotional, and spiritual care of self

    i) Delegates and supervises care responsibilities within the individual's scope of practice and/or other regulatory parameters

E. **Professional Growth and Development**

1. Maintain professional boundaries

    a) Understand team roles and work within them maintaining flexibility and willingness to blend roles as needed

    b) Set boundaries/limits for self and others in patient/family relationships

    c) Respond appropriately to those who overstep these boundaries

    d) Foster independence in patients and families

2. Provide self-care through stress management
    a) Assess self-care strategies
    b) Acknowledge potential stress/presence of stress
    c) Recognize ways to relieve stress
    d) Practice spiritual self-care
    e) Actively participate in stress management
    f) Seek assistance of others when indicated
    g) Maintain a balanced life
    h) Develop and maintain a strong support system
    i) Stay involved with the team dynamics for support and understanding

3. Participate in peer review and development
    a) Seek ways to precept, educate and mentor others
    b) Support and guide co-workers in clinical practice growth and development
    c) Accept the support of others
    d) Assist in developing mentoring programs

4. Commit to self-growth
    a) Commit to continuing education through journals, conferences, educational opportunities
    b) Commit to membership in professional specialty organizations and participate in the activities provided locally, regionally and nationally
    c) Participate and support research efforts to establish evidence based outcomes incorporating these outcomes into practice

F. **Mentor**[1,5]

1. Can be in a formal relationship such as orientation or informally as assistant
2. Individual having advanced knowledge and experience in an area of work who shares this knowledge with a newer team member
3. Mentors may not necessarily work side-by-side with the newer colleague, but are available to listen, support, and guide the newer colleague to become more familiar with the job and agency processes

G. **Networking**[1,5]

1. Communication with other hospice and palliative care team members
2. Allows for opportunity to share information about hospice and palliative care in general and particular cases with colleagues
3. May happen in a variety of settings (e.g., at lunch or in the report room, also at conferences and meetings)
4. Connections made between people of similar backgrounds

5. Provides opportunities to discuss similar problems and solutions; decreases feelings of isolation
6. On-line through Special Interest Group listservs and HPNA Discussion Group

H. Certification[1,5]

1. Professional recognition of hospice and palliative nursing knowledge through the successful completion of an examination
2. Process through which a professional group validates an individual's qualifications and knowledge in the specialized area of practice
3. The National Board for Certification of Hospice and Palliative Nurses (NBCHPN®) began certifying LP/VNs in September 2004. LP/VNs who are certified use the credential of CHPLN®
4. Hospice and palliative certification is separate from licensure and is voluntary. It is not required by law for practice
5. Recertification every four years maintains the credibility of this knowledge

I. Advocacy[1,5]

1. Process and act of representing the wishes, values, or concerns of another individual who may be less able to do so
2. Advocates must have knowledge of the person's wishes, etc. and be assertive in stating those wishes to others

J. Collaboration[1]

1. Working together with other individuals in a positive and effective manner where the combination of the knowledge and gifts of each individual in the group results in better outcomes for the patient and family
2. Requires open communication, mutual respect, and similar goals or mission

K. Quality Improvement[6]

1. A commitment and a systemic approach to improve every process in every part of an organization: goal is to exceed customer's (usually patient and family) expectations of care
2. Is a process to identify and solve problems with a goal to improve care and patient outcomes
3. Example of Quality Improvement (QI) Model: the Plan-Do-Check-Act (PDCA) Cycle: Steps[1,6–8]

    a) Plan: identify a problem (e.g., families' reluctance to give opioid pain medications); design an approach to solve problems or improve outcomes (e.g., work with team to teach staff to ask families why they are reluctant to give pain medication and to talk to the families about how pain medications work; assist team to develop a teaching sheet on opioid pain medications)

    b) Do: institute the change and collect information about the effect of the changes on practice and outcomes (e.g., work with team to determine use of opioid pain medications and levels of pain following changes)

c) Check: analyze the results (e.g., with team compare the use of opioid pain medication and pain levels before and after the change; did they decease, increase, or stay the same?)

d) Act: if the changes resulted in better outcomes, then plan ways to maintain the positive gains; if outcomes did not change or get worse, develop different ways to approach the problem and test these approaches (e.g., if staff education and teaching sheets did not work, the agency could develop a formal procedure for discussing opioid pain medication with families)

4. Research[1]

a) A systematic study or examination of a problem or question

b) Similar to QI, but usually more detailed

c) Research can take many forms: interviews, surveys, physical and chemical measures (e.g., blood pressure, pain, laboratory values)

d) Reported in professional journals and presentations

e) Create evidence based practice for clinical application

III. Professional Expectations and Development

A. Achieving and Maintaining Competency: Education and Training[1]

1. Licensed practical/vocational nurses must graduate from an education program approved by their state board of nursing

2. Licensed practical/vocational nurses must pass the NCLEX-PN®

3. Licensed practical/vocational nurses should complete specific in-services and competency evaluation for the licensed practical/vocational nurse in hospice and palliative care

4. Licensed practical/vocational nurses should participate in optional learning experiences to maintain expertise

a) Read professional journals, newsletters and websites

b) View educational videotapes

c) Attend classes on topics related to hospice and palliative care

5. Licensed practical/vocational nurses should maintain personal continuing education plan to update knowledge

a) Track attendance at conferences and meetings

b) List educational opportunities by title and presenter

c) Retain copies of handouts and number of hours attended

6. Licensed practical/vocational nurses are encouraged to continue their formal education in nursing and/or other professional disciplines. Programs to further education in nursing can include

a) Registered nursing (RN): after attending either a diploma program, associate degree program or bachelor's program, nurses must successfully complete the NCLEX-RN® to practice as an RN

   (1) Diploma programs: affiliated with a hospital and are around 24 months in length

   (2) Associate Degree programs (ADN): affiliated with community/junior colleges and are 2 years in length

   (3) Bachelor of Science in Nursing (BSN): affiliated with colleges and universities and are 4 years in length

   (4) RN to BSN: a program offered by some colleges and universities to facilitate the achievement of a bachelor's degree for RNs

b) Masters (MSN, MN)

   (1) Offered by numerous colleges and universities in many specialties to prepare nurses with BSNs to practice in advanced nursing roles. Length is usually at least 2 years, but depends on field of study. Examples can include

      i. Clinical nurse specialist: manages patient care at an advanced practice level

      ii. Nurse practitioner: delivers advanced practice nursing care independently

      iii. Education: preparation for teaching nurses in schools of nursing or staff development

c) Doctorate (PhD/DNP): offered by universities to prepare nurses with an MSN or MN to focus on research or practice

B. Mentoring[1,5]

1. Mentor other licensed practical/vocational nurses and nursing assistants in work place to share experiences and provide support and friendship

2. Help and participate in in-services, orientation, and other programs

3. Mentor student nurses, social worker and chaplain interns, medical students, and others

4. Precept new staff and provide guidance and support

5. Assist in the development and evaluation of preceptor/mentor programs

C. Networking and Professional Relationships[1,5]

1. Participate in membership organizations that promote quality nursing care (e.g., Hospice and Palliative Nurses Association)

2. Volunteer for committees at work and for professional organizations

3. Network with peers to share information and promote connectedness within the professional

D. Certification[1]

1. Certification assists in meeting professional expectations by providing educational, networking, mentoring and advocacy opportunities

2. Involves meeting eligibility requirements and passing a standardized test that reflects a national standard of knowledge needed to provide quality hospice and palliative licensed practical/vocational nursing care based on a test content outline

E. **Advocacy**[1]

1. Listen carefully to learn patients' and families' goals and values

2. Learn assertive communication skills to share patients' and families' goals with other team members

3. Remind team members and community about the importance of the licensed practical/vocational nurse in hospice and palliative care as a team member

4. Support fellow licensed practical/vocational nurses when they have good ideas about improving care of the seriously ill and dying

5. Volunteer/join local or regional groups that focus on quality care of the seriously ill and dying

F. **Quality Improvement (QI)**[1]

1. Licensed practical/vocational nurses should participate in QI activities at work; volunteer for the QI committee

    a) Provide ideas and feedback on agency processes and practices that could be improved to serve the patient and family

    b) Report problems or issues that have (or potentially have) a negative or harmful impact on patient, families, and staff

G. **Research**[1,5]

1. Licensed practical/vocational nurses should volunteer to gather data and information as directed by the research team

2. Licensed practical/vocational nurses should assist in using research findings in practice

3. Critical steps in research

    a) Develop an idea

    b) Define the problem/issue/question

    c) Collect background information

    d) Develop a written plan

    e) State objectives or hypotheses

    f) Determine research design

    g) Collect data

    h) Analyze data

    i) Draw conclusions

    j) Apply findings to clinical practice as appropriate

    k) Disseminate findings to colleagues

H. **Read Medical and Nursing Journals to Remain Current in Knowledge of treatment Options and End-of-Life Care**[5]

1. Peer reviewed: more formal articles with extensive literature reviews that are reviewed by content experts for accurateness before being published

    a) Research articles: peer reviewed article that is based on an individual or group research study

2. Non-peer reviewed: less formal articles based on personal opinion or experiences

I. **Participate in Professional Nursing Organization Activities**[5]

1. Hospice and Palliative Nurses Association (www.HPNA.org)

    a) National

    b) Chapters

2. State organizations

3. LP/VN organizations include

    a) National Association of Practical Nursing Education and Service, Inc. (www.napnes.org)

    b) National Federation of Licensed Practical Nurses, Inc. (www.nflpn.org)

4. Attend state and national conferences

5. Obtain certification in specialty areas of practice (i.e., hospice and palliative nursing)

J. **Participate in Peer Review**

1. Participate in peer review process according to agency's policies

K. **Maintain Professional Boundaries between Patients/Family and Staff**[5]

1. Understand team members' roles

2. Maintaining boundaries minimizes conflict

3. Work within defined role limits as appropriate, but be flexible, able and willing to blend roles when necessary

4. Each team member should be aware of need to set limits/boundaries for self and others when interacting with patients and families

5. Foster independence of patients and families; empower them to maintain maximum control of their lives

IV. **Addressing Professional Stresses**

A. **Sources of Stress for Professional Caregivers at the End of Life**[1]

1. Your own grief

2. Personal comfort level with dying

3. Feeling of helplessness
4. Sense that others do not care as much as you do
5. Lack of time to provide the care that you want to
6. Accept that stress exists and will be experienced by everyone who works with the dying and their families
7. Acknowledge that people often do not recognize stress in themselves

B. **Manifestations of Stress**[1]
1. Physical distress and fatigue
2. Feeling irritable a lot of the time
3. Emotional withdrawal from persons you are caring for
4. Trouble with personal relationships
5. Starting to feel like you are the only one who can give good care

C. **Interventions to Prevent and Decrease Job-Related Stress**[1,5]
1. Recognize that everyone on the team needs each other; no one is giving care alone
2. Start or maintain physical exercise program
3. Take care of your own emotional and spiritual needs
4. Find people with whom you feel comfortable talking to about feelings
5. Recognize that you cannot be or do everything for everyone; remember that even "Superman" is Clark Kent most of the time!
6. Be aware that clinical competency helps to reduce stress—take advantage of educational opportunities
7. Increase knowledge regarding palliative care, bereavement support and public policy affecting palliative care
8. Develop and maintain strong personal support systems
9. Maintain a balance in interactions with patients and families. Self-awareness is important in maintenance of appropriate boundaries
10. Secure a sense of closure after patients' deaths
11. Get adequate rest, eat a proper diet and participate in regular physical exercise
12. Remain involved with the team for mutual support and a feeling of belonging

D. **Advocate for the Profession**[5]
1. Keep informed about the state and federal policies that impact palliative care
2. Know and support various professional organizations' position statements on palliative care; maintain open dialogue on this topic
3. Educate policy makers, legislators about the needs of families experiencing palliative care

CITED REFERENCES

1. Sheldon JE, Poleto MA. Personal and professional development. In: Ersek M, ed. *Hospice and Palliative Nursing Assistant Core Curriculum*. Pittsburgh, PA: Hospice and Palliative Nurses Association; 2009:87–93.

2. National Board of Medical Examiners. *The Behaviors of Professionalism*. Available at: http://ci.nbme.org/professionalism/behaviors.asp. Accessed September 8, 2009.

3. Dahlin C, Lentz J, Sutermaster DJ. *Statement of the Scope and Standards of Hospice and Palliative Licensed Practical/Vocational Nursing Practice*. Dubuque, IA: Kendall Hunt Publishing; 2004.

4. Dahlin C, Lentz J, Sutermaster DJ. *Competencies for the Hospice and Palliative Licensed Practical/Vocational Nurse*. 2nd ed. Dubuque, IA: Kendall Hunt Publishing; 2009.

5. Owens D, Dockter D. Interdisciplinary collaborative practice in the hospice and palliative care setting. In: Berry P, ed. *Core Curriculum for the Generalist Hospice and Palliative Nurse*. Dubuque, IA: Kendall Hunt Publishing; 2005:15–21.

6. Bookbinder M. Improving the quality of care across all settings. In: Ferrell BR, Coyle N, eds. *Textbook of Palliative Nursing*. 2nd ed. New York, NY: Oxford University Press; 2006:725–757.

7. Deming WE. *Out of the Crisis*. Cambridge, MA: Massachusetts Institute of Technology Center for Advanced Engineering Study; 1986.

8. Nelson EC, Batalden PB, Ryer JC, eds. *Joint Commission Clinical Improvement Action Guide*. Oakbrook Terrace, IL: The Joint Accreditation of Healthcare Organizations; 1998.

ADDITIONAL REFERENCES AND RESOURCES

Cox S, Wener B, HPNA Board of Directors. Value of the licensed practical/vocational nurse in palliative care. *Journal of Hospice and Palliative Nursing*. 2009;11(2):129–130.

Duggleby W, Wright K. The hope of professional caregivers caring for persons at the end of life. *Journal of Hospice and Palliative Nursing*. 2007;9(1):42–49.

Perry B. Achieving professional fulfillment as a palliative care nurse. *Journal of Hospice and Palliative Nursing*. 2009;11(2):109–118.

Syme A, Bruce A. Hospice and palliative care: what unites us, what divides us? *Journal of Hospice and Palliative Nursing*. 2009;11(1):19–24.

Weigel C, Parker G, Fanning L, et al. Apprehension among hospital nurses providing end-of-life care. *Journal of Hospice and Palliative Nursing*. 2007;(2):86–91.

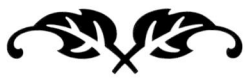

APPENDIX 1

WEBSITE/INTERNET RESOURCES[1]

Agency for Healthcare Research and Quality (AHRQ)	www.ahcpr.gov/
Aging with Dignity	www.agingwithdignity.org
The Alliance for Excellence in Hospice and Palliative Nursing	theallianceforexcellence.org
Alliance of State Pain Initiatives	www.aspi.wisc.edu
American Academy of Hospice and Palliative Medicine	www.aahpm.org
American Academy of Pain Medicine	www.painmed.org
American Association for Therapeutic Humor	www.aath.org
American Cancer Society	www.cancer.org
American Chronic Pain Association	www.theacpa.org/
American Headache Society	www.achenet.org
American Geriatrics Society	www.americangeriatrics.org
American Holistic Nurses Association	www.ahna.org
American Hospice Foundation	www.americanhospice.org
American Journal of Hospice and Palliative Medicine	ajh.sagepub.com/
American Journal of Nursing, Palliative Care Series	www.AJNonline.com
American Massage Therapy Association	www.amtamassage.org
American Nurses Association	www.nursingworld.org
American Pain Foundation	www.painfoundation.org
American Pain Society	www.ampainsoc.org
American Society for Bioethics and Humanities	www.asbh.org
American Society of Anesthesiologists	www.asahq.org
American Society of Clinical Oncology (ASCO)	www.asco.org
American Society of Law, Medicine and Ethics	www.aslme.org
American Society of Pain Management Nursing	www.aspmn.org
Americans for Better Care of the Dying	www.abcd-caring.org/
Approaching Death: Improving Care at the End of Life	www.nap.edu/readingroom/books/approaching/

[1] Adapted in part from Virani R, Garcia L. Palliative care resource list. In: Ferrell BR, Coyle N, eds. *Textbook of Palliative Nursing.* 3rd ed. New York, NY: Oxford University Press, Inc.; 2010.

Arthritis Foundation	www.arthritis.org
Association for Death Education and Counseling (ADEC)	www.adec.org
Association of Cancer Online Resources, Inc.	www.acor.org
Association of Nurses in AIDS Care	www.anacnet.org
Association of Oncology Social Work (AOSW)	www.aosw.org
Association of Pediatric Hematology/Oncology Nurses (APON)	www.apon.org
Before I Die: Medical Care and Personal Choices	www.thirteen.org/bid
Cancer Care®	www.cancercare.org
CancerLink	www.personal.u-net.com/~njh/cancer.html
Candlelighters Childhood Cancer Foundation	www.candlelighters.org
Caregiver Network	www.ltcplanningnetwork.com
Catholic Health Association of the United States	www.chausa.org
Center for Disease Control and Prevention	www.cdc.gov
Center for Palliative Care	www.hms.harvard.edu/cdi/pallcare
Center to Advance Palliative Care	www.capc.org
Children's Hospice International	www.chionline.org
Choices	www.choices.org
City of Hope Pain/Palliative Care Resource Center	prc.coh.org
The Compassionate Friends Inc.	www.compassionatefriends.org/
Compassion in Dying Federation	www.compassionandchoices.org
ConsultGeriRN.org	consultgerirn.org/
Dying Well	www.dyingwell.org
Education in Palliative and End-of-Life Care (EPEC)	www.epec.net
The End of Life: Exploring Death in America	www.npr.org/programs/death/
End of Life/Palliative Education Resource Center (EPERC)	www.eperc.mcw.edu
End-of-Life Nursing Education Consortium (ELNEC)	www.aacn.nche.edu/ELNEC
European Association for Palliative Care (EAPC)	www.eapcnet.org
The European Journal of Palliative Care	www.ejpc.eu.com
Family Caregiver Alliance®	www.caregiver.org
Fibromyalgia Network	www.fmnetnews.com
GeroNurse Online	www.geronurseonline.org
Grief.Net	www.griefnet.org
Growth House, Inc.	www.growthhouse.org
Hospice and Palliative Nurses Association	www.hpna.org
Hospice and Palliative Nurses Foundation	www.hpnf.org
Hospice Foundation of America (HFA)	www.hospicefoundation.org
Hospice Net	www.hospicenet.org
Hospice Resources.Net	www.hospiceresources.net

Institute for Healthcare Improvement	www.ihi.org
International Association for Hospice and Palliative Care	www.hospicecare.com
International Association for the Study of Pain®	www.iasp-pain.org/
International Journal of Palliative Nursing	www.ijpn.co.uk/
The International Workgroup on Death, Dying, and Bereavement	www.chernydatabase.org/
Journal of Pain and Palliative Care Pharmacotherapy	www.haworthpress.com
Journal of Pain and Symptom Management	www.elsevier.com
Journal of Palliative Care	www.ircm.qc.ca/bioethique/english
Journal of Palliative Medicine	www.liebertpub.com/products/product.aspx?pid=41
Journal of the American College of Surgeons, Palliative Care in Surgery Series	www.facs.org/cqi/jacarticles.hetm
Leukemia & Lymphoma Society®	www.leukemia.org
Long Term Care Planning Network	www.ltcplanningnetwork.com
Make a Wish Foundation®	www.wish.org
Memorial Sloan-Kettering Cancer Center	www.mskcc.org
The Nathan Cummings Foundation	www.sicklecelldisease.org
National Association for Home Care and Hospice (NAHC)	www.nahc.org/
National Board for Certification of Hospice and Palliative Nurses	www.nbchpn.org
National Cancer Institute Cancer Topics	www.cancer.gov/cancerinformation
National Comprehensive Cancer Network (NCCN)	www.nccn.org/
National Conference of State Legislatures	www.ncsl.org/programs/pubs/endoflife.htm
National Consensus Project for Quality Palliative Care	www.nationalconsensusproject.org
National Family Caregivers Association	www.nfcacares.org/
National Hospice and Palliative Care Organization	www.nhpco.org
The National Institute on Aging	www.nih.gov/nia/
National Prison Hospice Association	www.npha.org
National Quality Forum (NQF) Framework for Preferred Practices for Palliative and Hospice Care	www.qualityforum.org/Topics/Palliative_and_End-of-Life_Care.aspx
The Neuropathy Association	www.neuropathy.org
Not Dead Yet	www.notdeadyet.org/
On Our Own Terms	www.pbs.org/wnet/onourownterms/
OncoLink	www.oncolink.com
Oncology Nursing Society	www.ons.org
Open Society Institute	www.soros.org
Oregon Health Sciences University Center for Ethics in Health Care	www.ohsu.edu/ethics/
PainLink	www.edc.org/PainLink
Palliative & Supportive Care	journals.cambridge.org/action/displayJournal?jid=PAX

Palliative Care Policy Center	www.medicaring.org
Palliative Medicine	Pmj.sagepub.com
Partners Against Pain®	www.partnersagainstpain.com
Patient Education Institute	www.patient-education.com
Progress in Palliative Care	www.ingentaconnect.com/content/maney/ppc
Promoting Excellence in End-of-Life Care	www.promotingexcellence.org
Reflex Sympathetic Dystrophy Association of California	www.rsdsa-ca.org/
Regional Palliative Care Program in Edmonton Alberta	www.palliative.org
The Robert Wood Johnson Foundation	www.rwjf.org
Shaare Zedek Cancer Pain and Palliative Care Reference Database	www.chernydatabase.org/
Sickle Cell Disease Association of America, Inc.	www.sicklecelldisease.org
Southern California Cancer Pain Initiative (SCCPI)	sccpi.coh.org
Supportive Care Coalition	www.supportivecarecoalition.org
Take Charge of Your Life	www.takechargeonline.org/
Task Force on Life & the Law: When Death is Sought	www.health.state.ny.us/nysdoh/provider/death.htm
Telemedicine Information Exchange	tie.telemed.org
TMJ Association, Ltd.	www.tmj.org
Today's Caregiver	www.caregiver.com/
U. S. Department of Health and Human Services, Healthfinder®	www.healthfinder.gov
UNIPAC Series	www.liebertpub.com/products/product.aspx?pid=119
United Hospital Fund of New York	www.uhfnyc.org
University of Wisconsin Pain & Policy Studies Group	www.wisc.edu
VistaCare	www.vista-care.com
World Health Organization	www.who.int/en

Editor's Note: Any URLs found to be non-functional or inaccurate at the time of publication have been either corrected or deleted.

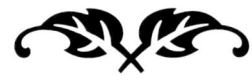

APPENDIX 2

COMMONLY USED MEDICATIONS
Trade and Generic Names Medication Class[1]

ANTICHOLINESTERASE (used for the treatment of dementia of the Alzheimer's type)
Aricept®	donepezil
Cognex®	tacrine
Exelon®	rivastigmine
Namenda®	memantine
Reminyl®	galantamine

ANALGESICS
Actiq®	fentaNYL* citrate
AVINza®*/Kadian®/MS Contin®/ Oramorph® SR/Roxanol®	morphine sulfate
Dilaudid®/Palladone™	HYDROmorphone*
Dolophine®	methadone
Duragesic®	fentaNYL* transdermal system
Tylenol w/Codeine®	acetaminophen/codeine
Fiorinal®	aspirin/caffeine/butalbital
Lidoderm HCL Topical®	lidocaine
Levo-Dromoran®	levorphanol
OxyContin®*/OxyFAST®	oxyCODONE*
Percocet®/Roxicet®	oxyCODONE*/acetaminophen
Percodan®	oxyCODONE*/aspirin
Tylenol®	acetaminophen
Ultram®	traMADol*
Vicodin®/Lorcet®	HYDROcodone*/acetaminophen

ANTACIDS/ANTIFLATULENTS/DIGESTANTS
Basaljel®	aluminum carbonate gel
Carafate®	sucralfate
Maalox®	magnesium hydroxide/aluminum hydroxide
Mylanta®	magnesium hydroxide/aluminum hydroxide/simethicone
Mylicon®	simethicone
Pancrease®/Viokase®	pancrelipase

ANTIANGINAL
Calan®/Isoptin®	verapamil
Isordil®	isosorbide dinitrate

Cardizem®	diltiazem
Persantine®	dipyridamole
Procardia®	NIFEdipine*

ANTIBIOTICS

Ancef®	ceFAZolin*
Augmentin®	amoxicillin/clavulanate
Bactrim®	trimethoprim/sulfamethoxazole
Biaxin®	clarithromycin
Ceclor®	cefaclor
Cefobid®	cefoperazone
Ceftin®	cefuroxime
Claforan®	cefotaxime
Cleocin®	clindamycin
Fortaz®	ceftazidime
Garamycin®	gentamicin
Rocephin®	cefTRIAXone*
Timentin®	ticarcillin/clavulanate
Unasyn®	ampicillin/sulbactam
Zithromax®	azithromycin
Zosyn®	piperacillin/tazobactam

ANTICOAGULANTS

Coumadin®	warfarin
Lovenox®	enoxaparin

ANTICONVULSANTS

Depacon®	valproate
Depakote®	valproic acid
Dilantin®	phenytoin
Keppra®	levetiracetam
KlonoPIN®*	clonazepam
LaMICtal®*	lamoTRIgine*
Mysoline®	primidone
Neurontin®	gabapentin
TEGretol®*	carBAMazepine*
Topamax®	topiramate
Zonegran®	zonisamide
Lyrica®	pregabalin

ANTIDEPRESSANTS

Adapin®/Sinequan®	doxepin
CeleXA®*	citalopram
Cymbalta®	DULoxetine*
Desyrel®	traZODone*
Effexor®	venlafaxine
Elavil®/Endep®	amitriptyline
Lexapro®	escitalopram
Luvox®	fluvoxamine
Norpramin®	desipramine
Pamelor®	nortriptyline

Paxil®	PARoxetine*
PROzac®*	FLUoxetine*
Remeron®	mirtazapine
Serzone®	nefazodone
Surmontil®	trimipramine
Tofranil®	imipramine
Tofranil® PM	imipramine pamoate
Vivactil®	protriptyline
Wellbutrin®	buPROPion*
Zoloft®	sertraline

ANTIDIABETES

Amaryl®	glimepiride
Glucotrol®/Glucotrol XL®	glipiZIDE*
Glynase®/Micronase®	glyBURIDE*
Glucophage®	metFORMIN*
Prandin®	repaglinide
Starlix®	nateglinide

ANTIDIARRHEAL

Donnagel®/Kaopectate®	kaolin/pectin
Imodium®	loperamide
Lomotil®	diphenoxylate/atropine
Pepto-Bismol®	bismuth subsalicylate
Paregoric®	camphorated opium tincture
Sandostatin®	octreotide

ANTIFUNGALS

Diflucan®	fluconazole
Flagyl®	metroNIDAZOLE*
Monistat®	miconazole nitrate
Mycelex®/Lotrimin®	clotrimazole
Nizoral®	ketoconazole
Mycostatin®	nystatin
Sporanox®	itraconazole

ANTIGOUT

Benemid®	probenecid
Zyloprim®/Lopurin®	allopurinol

ANTIHYPERTENSIVES

Catapres®	cloNIDine*
Capoten®	captopril
Corgard®	nadolol
Inderal®	propranolol
Lopressor®	metoprolol
Prinivil®/Zestril®	lisinopril
Tenormin®	atenolol
Trandate®	labetalol
Vasotec®	enalapril
Norvasc®	amLODIPine*

ANTIHISTAMINES
Allegra®	fexofenadine
Atarax®	hydrOXYzine*
Benadryl®	diphenhydrAMINE*
Chlor-Trimeton®	chlorpheniramine
Clarinex®	desloratadine
Claritin®/Alavert®	loratadine
Tavist®	clemastine
ZyrTEC®*	cetirizine

ANTINAUSEA/ANTIEMETIC/ PROMOTILITY
Aloxi®	palonosetron
Antivert®	meclizine
Anzemet®	dolasetron
Compazine®	prochlorperazine
Dramamine®	dimenhyDRINATE*
Emend®	aprepitant
Haldol®	haloperidol
Kytril®	granisetron
Phenergan®	promethazine
Reglan®	metoclopramide
Thorazine®	chlorproMAZINE*
Tigan®	trimethobenzamide
Torecan®	thiethylperazine
Trilafon®	perphenazine
Zofran®	ondansetron

ANTIPARKINSON AGENTS
Apokyn®	apomorphine
Artane®	trihexyphenidyl
Cogentin®	benztropine
Mirapex®	pramipexole
Parlodel®	bromocriptine
Permax®	pergolide
Sinemet®	carbidopa/levodopa
Stalevo®	carbidopa/levodopa/entacapone
Symmetrel®	amantadine

ANTIPRURITICS
Caladryl®	calamine/diphenhydrAMINE*

ANTIPSYCHOTICS
Clozaril®	clozapine
Haldol®	haloperidol
Loxitane®	loxapine
Mellaril®	thioridazine
Moban®	molindone
Navane®	thiothixene
Prolixin®	fluphenazine
Risperdal®	risperidone
SEROquel®*	QUEtiapine*

Stelazine®	trifluoperazine
Thorazine®	chlorproMAZINE*
Trilafon®	perphenazine
ZyPREXA®*	OLANZapine

ANTISECRETORY/ANTICHOLINERGICS
Levsin®	hyoscyamine
Transderm-Scop®	scopolamine

ANTIVIRAL
Famvir®	famciclovir
Valtrex®	valacyclovir
Zovirax®	acyclovir

ANXIOLYTIC/ANTIDEPRESSANT
Etrafon®/Triavil®	perphenazine/amitriptyline

ANXIOLYTIC/SEDATIVES
Ambien®	zolpidem
Ativan®	LORazepam*
Zydis®/Zyprexa®	olanzapine
BuSpar®	busPIRone
Dalmane®	flurazepam
Halcion®	triazolam
Klonopin®	clonazePAM*
Librium®	chlordiazePOXIDE*
Placidyl®	ethchlorvynol
Restoril®	temazepam

APPETITE STIMULANTS
Megace®	megestrol

BISPHOSPHONATES
Aredia®	pamidronate
Zometa®	zoledronic acid
Fosamax®	alendronate

CARDIAC GLYCOSIDES
Lanoxin®	digoxin

H_2 BLOCKERS/PROTON PUMP INHIBITORS
NexIUM®*	esomeprazole
Pepcid®	famotidine
Prevacid®	lansoprazole
PriLOSEC®*	omeprazole
Protonix®	pantoprazole
Tagamet®	cimetidine
Zantac®	ranitidine

LAXATIVES
Benefiber®	soluble fiber
CitroMag®	magnesium citrate

Citrucel®	methylcellulose
Chronulac®	lactulose
Colace®/Surfak®/Regutol®	docusate sodium
Dulcolax®	bisacodyl
Fiberall®/FiberCon®	calcium polycarbophil
Fleet Enema®	sodium biphosphate/phosphate
Metamucil®	psyllium
MiraLax™	polyethylene glycol
Phillips' Milk of Magnesia®	magnesium hydroxide
Senokot®	senna
Serax®	oxazepam
Sonata®	zaleplon
Tranxene®	clorazepate
Valium®	diazepam
Versed®	midazolam

MUSCLE RELAXANTS

Flexeril®	cyclobenzaprine
Lioresal®	baclofen
Norflex®	orphenadrine
Robaxin®	methocarbamol
Soma®	carisoprodol
Quinamm®	quinine sulfate
Valium, Valrelease®	diazepam

NSAIDs

Aleve®/Anaprox®/Naprosyn®	naproxen sodium
CeleBREX®*	celecoxib
Indocin®	indomethacin
Motrin®	ibuprofen
Trilisate®	choline magnesium trisalicylate

PSYCHOSTIMULANTS

Dexedrine®	dextroamphetamine
Provigil®	modafinil
Ritalin®	methylphenidate

CORTICOSTEROIDS

Decadron®	dexamethasone
Deltasone®	predniSONE*
Orapred®/Prelone®	prednisoLONE*
Medrol®/Solu-Medrol®	methylPREDNISolone*
Solu-Cortef®	hydrocortisone

"Tall man" (mixed case) lettering is used, as suggested by the FDA, Institute for Safe Medication Practices (ISMP), and the Joint Commission, to differentiate look-alike medication names from one another.[2]

Cited References

1. Medline Plus, Drugs, Supplements, and Herbal Information. Available at: http://www.nlm.nih.gov/medlineplus/druginformation.html. Accessed December 30, 2009.
2. Institute for Safe Medication Practices (ISMP). *FDA and ISMP Lists of Look-Alike Drug Name Sets With Recommended Tall Man Letters.* 2008. Available at: http://www.ismp.org/tools/tallmanletters.pdf. Accessed December 30, 2009.

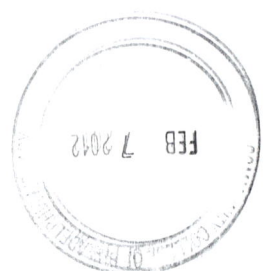